Small Animal Ophthalmology

Small Animal Ophthalmology

What's Your Diagnosis?

Heidi Featherstone BVetMed DVOphthal DipECVO MRCVS

Willows Veterinary Centre and Referral Service

Solihull, West Midlands, UK

Elaine Holt DVM DipACVO DipECVO MRCVS

North Downs Specialist Referrals

Bletchingley, Surrey, UK

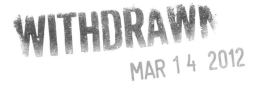

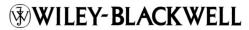

WILEY-BLACKWELL

A John Wiley & Sons, Ltd., Publication

This edition first published 2011 by Blackwell Publishing Ltd

© 2011 by Heidi Featherstone and Elaine Holt

Blackwell Publishing was acquired by John Wiley & Sons in February 2007. Blackwell's publishing program has been merged with Wiley's global Scientific, Technical and Medical business to form Wiley-Blackwell.

Registered office: John Wiley & Sons Ltd, The Atrium, Southern Gate, Chichester, West Sussex, PO19 8SQ, UK

Editorial offices: 9600 Garsington Road, Oxford, OX4 2DQ, UK

The Atrium, Southern Gate, Chichester, West Sussex, PO19 8SQ, UK

2121 State Avenue, Ames, Iowa 50014-8300, USA

For details of our global editorial offices, for customer services and for information about how to apply for permission to reuse the copyright material in this book please see our website at www.wiley.com/wiley-blackwell.

Library of Congress Cataloging-in-Publication Data

Featherstone, Heidi

  Small animal ophthalmology : what's your diagnosis? / Heidi Featherstone, Elaine Holt.

      p. ; cm.

  Includes bibliographical references and index.

  ISBN 978-1-4051-5161-0 (pbk. : alk. paper)

  1. Veterinary ophthalmology.   2. Pet medicine.   I. Holt, Elaine.   II. Title.

  [DNLM: 1. Eye Diseases–veterinary–Case Reports.   2. Eye Diseases–veterinary–Problems and Exercises.

  3. Animals, Domestic–Case Reports.   4. Animals, Domestic–Problems and Exercises.   5. Diagnosis, Differential–Case

  Reports.   6. Diagnosis, Differential–Problems and Exercises. SF 891]

    SF891.F43 2011

    636.089'77–dc22

                            2010041328

A catalogue record for this book is available from the British Library.

This book is published in the following electronic formats: ePDF 9781444340013; ePub 9781444340020

Set in 10/12.5 pt MinionPro by Toppan Best-set Premedia Limited
Printed and bound in Malaysia by Vivar Printing Sdn Bhd

1   2011

Contents

Foreword

Welcome to one of the most useful and informative ophthalmology text-books to have been published in recent years. The authors are to be commended on creating a reference book that is unlike any other currently on the market. They are medical educators that have drawn from a wealth of private practice knowledge and experience to create a highly practical guide to some of the most common presentations of ophthalmic disease. This highly utilitarian and functional approach is exemplified by their overall organizational approach. Rather than assuming the traditional 'front to back' approach taught in most classroom settings, the purpose of this text can be first best reflected in its chapters' titles, whereby they encompass the most frequently encountered small animal patient complaints such as ocular discharge, the painful eye, the opaque eye, the abnormal pupil, blindness, and ocular trauma (to name just a few). The strength of this textbook is evident that all major topic areas have been presented using actual cases, which are both beautifully photodocumented and carefully organized. In addition to the numerous high quality coloured photographs, are clear illustrations, the results of advanced imaging modalities which in some cases utilize 3D reconstruction, and histopathology – all which dramatically strengthen the calibre of each case presentation.

The book will appeal to veterinary clinicians at all stages of the educational process, ranging from veterinary students and new graduates to board-certified ophthalmic specialists. The employment of case-based examples prompts the reader to hone his/her clinical acumen by working through relevant questions pertaining to differential diagnoses and the selection of appropriate diagnostic tests. Diagnosis, treatment, prognosis, and discussion are clearly provided. Importantly, the authors recognize that, depending on the reader's level of experience, different diagnostic and therapeutic strategies may, at times, be equally successful to those provided and thus ample opportunities for additional reading is provided by way of several appendices, glossaries, and extensive bibliographic material. As I have, I believe you will find this text one of the most enjoyable, informative, and 'user-friendly' practical approaches to small animal ophthalmology to have been published in many years.

Elizabeth A. Giuliano, DVM, MS
Diplomate, American College of Veterinary Ophthalmologists

Preface

Veterinary ophthalmology is a visual discipline – not because the eye is the organ of vision but because the evidence that is required to diagnose ocular disease in animals is often highly visible. In other veterinary specialities a problem typically requires extensive investigation, but in veterinary ophthalmology a thorough ocular examination and a few routine tests may well result in an accurate diagnosis. The challenge is to know what to look for, and then to interpret the clinical signs correctly. Techniques such as electroretinography and advanced diagnostic imaging have their place, but only in a small number of cases.

There are numerous textbooks in both the human and veterinary fields containing comprehensive information on all aspects of ophthalmology, from anatomy and physiology to the treatment of clinical disease. The aim of this book is to offer the reader a practical guide to diagnosis using a case-based, systematic approach. It is intended for anyone with an interest in veterinary ophthalmology, including the general practitioner and the veterinary student.

We are veterinary ophthalmologists working in busy referral practices, with experience in general practice and in undergraduate and postgraduate teaching. We have sought to provide a pragmatic approach to the diagnosis and management of ocular disease in small animals, and to share our thought processes, drawing on the broad spectrum of examples in our daily case loads, from extreme forms of common conditions to more complex ocular disease. Practical recommendations are supported by extensive photodocumentation, and an appendix of tips for interpreting the information obtained from ophthalmic examination.

Heidi Featherstone & Elaine Holt

Acknowledgements

As with any book, the finished work is possible only with the help of many people. We are indebted to numerous colleagues, not only for generously contributing case material, but also for their time and advice. For their ophthalmology expertise, we thank Peter Renwick, Christine Heinrich, John Mould, Mike Rhodes, Barbara Braus, Sue Manning, Elizabeth Giuliano, Ellison Bentley, Marnie Ford and David Gould. Peter Renwick and Christine Heinrich deserve special thanks for their generosity in sharing their library of photographs, built up over many years. John Mould also deserves special thanks for his exceptional photographic skills, and for his readiness to share his photographs. With respect to imaging, we are grateful to Paul Mahoney for his tireless help and advice on advanced imaging techniques, and to Ruth Dennis and Rob White for sharing their case material. Emma Scurrell has provided invaluable expertise, along with enthusiasm, on ophthalmic pathology, supported by excellent gross and histological photographs. Simon Scurrell has worked skilfully and painstakingly on the annotated diagrams. Photographing the eyes of conscious dogs and cats is a challenge that requires excellent handling skills and patience: special thanks to David Hindley, Stephanie Ascott, Tom Buckley, Nicola Millington, Lou Hadley and the nursing team at Willows Veterinary Centre and Referral Service. Sue Jenkins' non-veterinary editing expertise has been invaluable throughout.

Not least, we would like to thank the animals, their owners, and the referring veterinary surgeons, without whom this book would not have been possible.

List of Abbreviations

ACTH	adrenocorticotrophic hormone (adrenocorticotropin)
ALT	alanine aminotransferase
AP	alkaline phosphatase
CCT	corneoconjunctival transposition
CDV	canine distemper virus
CNS	central nervous system
CT	computed tomography
CTT	corneal touch threshold
DIM	diffuse iris melanoma
EOM	extraocular polymyositis
ERG	electroretinography
FCV	feline calicivirus
FeLV	feline leukaemia virus
FHV-1	feline herpesvirus-1
FIV	feline immunodeficiency virus
FNA	fine-needle aspiration
H&E	haematoxylin and eosin
HF-UBM	high-frequency ultrasound biomicroscopy
ICLE	intracapsular lens extraction
IMR	immune-mediated retinitis
IOP	intraocular pressure
IVIg	intravenous therapy with human immunoglobulin
KCS	keratoconjunctivitis sicca
LIU	lens-induced uveitis
MMM	masticatory muscle myositis
MRI	magnetic resonance imaging
Nd:YAG	neodymium-doped yttrium aluminium garnet
NGE	nodular granulomatous episclerokeratitis
NSAID	non-steroidal anti-inflammatory drug
OD	oculus dextor, right eye
OS	oculus sinister, left eye

OU	oculi unitas, both eyes
PCR	polymerase chain reaction
PDT	parotid duct transposition
PHPV	persistent hyperplastic primary vitreous
PLR	pupillary light reflex
PPM	persistent pupillary membrane
PRA	progressive retinal atrophy
prcd	progressive rod-cone degeneration
q	quisque, every, e.g. q4 hours means 'every four hours' (six times daily)
RPE	retinal pigment epithelium
RPED	RPE dystrophy
SARDS	sudden acquired retinal degeneration syndrome
SFT	swinging flashlight test
STT	Schirmer tear test
TEL	third eyelid
TBUT	tear film break-up time
TPA	tissue plasminogen activator
UBM	ultrasound biomicroscopy
VOR	vestibulo-ocular reflex

CHAPTER 1

Abnormalities of Globe Size and Position

Introduction

It can be a challenge to differentiate between a change in size and a change in position of the eye. An abnormally small eye (microphthalmos) may be confused with a normal-sized eye that is recessed in the orbit (enophthalmos); an enlarged eye (buphthalmos) may have a similar appearance to a normal-sized eye that is anteriorly displaced (exophthalmos). Assessing the size of the palpebral fissure, position of the third eyelid (TEL) and corneal diameter, looking at the eye from different angles, careful comparison with the other eye and concurrent clinical signs are helpful in differentiating between these conditions.

Small Animal Ophthalmology: What's Your Diagnosis? First Edition. Heidi Featherstone, Elaine Holt.
© 2011 by Heidi Featherstone and Elaine Holt. Published 2011 by Blackwell Publishing Ltd.

History

A 12-year-old female neutered domestic shorthaired cat is presented because of a sudden redness in the right eye. The left eye had looked abnormal for several weeks but appeared comfortable. The cat has recently lost weight and is lethargic.

Questions

1. Describe the abnormalities in Figs. 1.1a, b, and c.
2. What differential diagnoses should be considered for this presentation?
3. What tests could you perform to make the diagnosis?

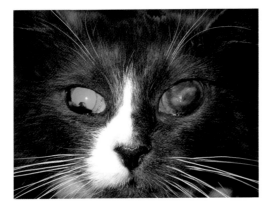

Fig. 1.1a

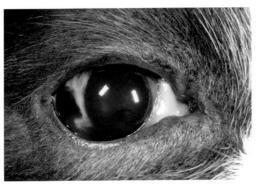

Fig. 1.1b

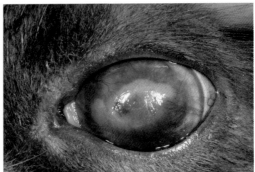

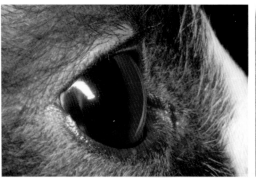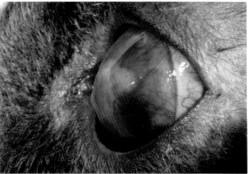

Fig. 1.1c

Answers

1. What the figures show
Fig. 1.1a The left eye appears larger than the right eye; a wide palpebral fissure, increased corneal diameter and clearly visible medial and lateral regions of the limbus are consistent with buphthalmos. There is a generalised corneal opacity which is most dense axially; a tapetal reflection is not visible. In the right eye, the green tapetal reflection is obstructed ventrally by a red/black irregular opacity which appears to be in front of the iris, and there is a similar coloured opacity overlying the iris at the 9 o'clock position. The pupil is moderately dilated.

Fig. 1.1b In the left eye, the Purkinje images are disrupted. There is generalised corneal vascularisation and a stippled area of fluorescein stain uptake axially. The conjunctival vessels overlying the sclera on the lateral aspect of the globe are congested. The iris is difficult to see well but appears darker (medially) and possibly thickened. In the right eye, there is hyphaema; the regions of the iris that are visible appear normal.

Fig. 1.1c Oblique view from the lateral aspect of both eyes. In the left eye there is an irregular contour and anterior protrusion of the cornea (OS > OD). There is increased exposure of the sclera and conjunctiva, and episcleral congestion. The anterior chamber is obliterated by abnormal iris tissue which appears to be displaced anteriorly. In both eyes fluorescein dye is visible on the periocular hair at the medial canthus.

2. Differential diagnoses
Given the history and the appearance of the left eye, the following conditions should be considered:

- **Chronic glaucoma** In contrast to the dog, primary glaucoma in the cat is rare, and secondary glaucoma is more common. The most common causes of secondary glaucoma in the cat are chronic idiopathic lymphocytic-plasmacytic uveitis and primary intraocular neoplasia, most notably diffuse iris melanoma. Typical clinical signs include buphthalmos, conjunctival and episcleral congestion, corneal oedema, mydriasis, and impaired or absent vision. Buphthalmos can be difficult to discern in the cat and assessment of the size of the palpebral fissure can be helpful because it becomes wider as the size of the eye increases. Glaucoma in cats is typically insidious in onset and is often difficult to recognise. This is in contrast to canine primary glaucoma which is characterised by peracute pain, episcleral congestion, marked corneal oedema, mydriasis and blindness (*Ch. 6, case 2*).

- **Exophthalmos** Anterior displacement of the globe within the orbit. Common causes of exophthalmos in the cat include orbital neoplasia, orbital cellulitis/abscess and orbital trauma

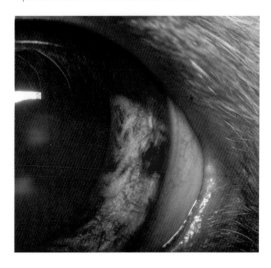

Fig. 1.1d Aneurysm within the lateral region of the major arterial circle in the left eye of a cat with systemic hypertension.

(haematoma, emphysema, fracture, foreign body). Primary malignant neoplasia and abscesses secondary to dental disease are more likely in old cats, whereas head trauma and orbital foreign bodies are more common in young cats (*Ch.12, case 2*).

Given the appearance of the right eye, the following conditions should be considered:

- **Systemic hypertension** Sustained systemic hypertension is commonly associated with ocular manifestations which primarily involve the posterior segment but also affect the anterior segment. Abnormalities in the posterior segment involve the retina, choroid and vitreous humour and appear as retinal oedema and bullae, retinal and intravitreal haemorrhages, retinal detachment and increased tortuosity of the retinal arterioles. Intraocular haemorrhage can occur as a result of haemorrhage from the iris (Fig. 1.1d), ciliary body, retina, and choroid. Extensive hyphaema can lead to the formation of anterior and posterior synechiae and secondary glaucoma.
- **Coagulopathy and platelet disorders** Ocular haemorrhage can be a clinical sign of a coagulopathy or a platelet disorder. Ocular haemorrhage typically occurs when the platelet count is <50 000 cells/μl.
- **Uveitis** When there is a breakdown of the blood-aqueous barrier during inflammation, red blood cells can enter the anterior chamber (hyphaema). The blood may form either a homogenous layer in the ventral anterior chamber or a clot, as in this cat.
- **Trauma** Ocular haemorrhage may result from both blunt and penetrating ocular trauma (*Ch. 12, cases 2 and 3*).
- **Pre-iridal fibrovascular membrane (PIFM)** The formation of fibrovascular membranes on the anterior iris is usually a consequence of intraocular inflammation, haemorrhage and/or hypoxia due to the release of vasoactive substances. Hence the formation of PIFMs is common in eyes with chronic uveitis, intraocular haemorrhage, retinal detachment, glaucoma, and neoplasia. The newly formed blood vessels within the membranes are fragile and can cause spontaneous and recurrent hyphaema. PIFMs can extend into the filtration angle and result in secondary glaucoma. Fibrovascular membranes are not restricted to the surface of the iris – they can also form on the retina and optic disc and in the vitreous.
- **Neoplasia (primary or secondary)** Intraocular haemorrhage may occur in eyes affected with primary or secondary neoplasia, either originating from a PIFM or as a result of the direct effect of neoplasia (e.g. adverse effect on clotting function).
- **Congenital anomalies** These include persistent hyaloid artery and persistent hyperplastic primary vitreous, both of which are rare conditions in the cat.

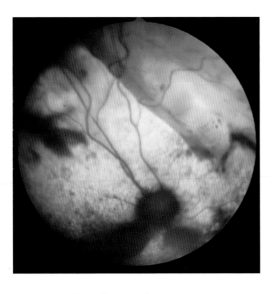

Fig. 1.1e Extensive dorsal retinal detachment and multiple retinal haemorrhages throughout the tapetal fundus and ventral to the optic disc.

3. Appropriate diagnostic tests

- Ocular reflexes
    - Pupillary light reflex – the left pupil is not visible. Negative consensual OS (from left to right eye); positive direct OD, albeit slow and incomplete.
    - Dazzle reflex – negative OS, positive OD
    - Palpebral reflex – positive OU, OS < OD
    - Corneal reflex – positive OU, OS < OD
- Menace response – negative OS, equivocal OD

In this cat, these results are consistent with blindness, reduced corneal sensation and lagophthalmos in the left eye, and reduced vision in the right eye.

- Examination with a focal light source – in the left eye, slit-lamp biomicroscopy reveals extensive superficial and deep corneal vascularisation, and generalised corneal oedema and fibrosis which is most marked axially.
- Ophthalmoscopy – in the right eye, this reveals an extensive dorsal retinal detachment, most marked within the medial quadrant, and multiple retinal haemorrhages of different sizes throughout the tapetal fundus and ventral to the optic disc (Fig. 1.1e).
- Schirmer tear test – 4 mm/min OS, 10 mm/min OD
- Fluorescein dye – negative staining OD, positive staining in the superficial axial cornea OS. This is indicative of suboptimal ocular surface health in the left eye, most likely because of the lagophthalmos.
- Tonometry – IOP 35 mmHg OS, 20 mmHg OD

There is increased resistance to retropulsion of the left eye; retropulsion of the right eye is normal. The remainder of the ophthalmic examination reveals no additional abnormalities. A general physical examination reveals an underweight body condition and mild dental disease.

> The degree of resistance to retropulsion of the eye varies amongst species and between breeds. The normal feline globe is generally retropulsed less than the normal canine globe because of close apposition between the globe and the orbit in the cat. The degree of retropulsion in brachycephalic breeds is less than in other breeds because of the shallow orbit, in both cats and dogs.

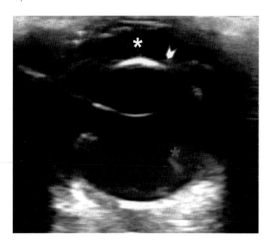

Fig. 1.1f Horizontal B-mode ultrasound scan (left eye). There is hyperechoic material spanning the anterior chamber (white asterix) and within the vitreous body (blue asterix); convex iris leaflets contact the anterior surface of the lens (arrow). In this cat, these changes are consistent with intraocular haemorrhage, anterior synechiae, and iris bombé.

Further diagnostic tests

- B-mode ocular ultrasound – this is indicated to evaluate the posterior segment when the anterior segment is opaque, and to take measurements. Axial globe length is the distance between the centre of the cornea and the posterior pole.

   The ultrasound scan reveals an axial globe length of 22 mm OS and 19 mm OD (within normal limits), which confirms buphthalmos in the left eye. Additional abnormalities in the left eye include hyperechoic material spanning the anterior chamber (consistent with blood, fibrin or anterior synechiae), hyperechoic material within the vitreous (consistent with vitreal degeneration, intravitreal haemorrhage, neoplasm), and convex iris leaflets which contact the anterior lens capsule (consistent with iris bombé, *Ch. 9, case 4*) (Fig. 1.1f).
- Laboratory tests – results of routine haematology, biochemistry (including electrolytes), urine analysis and thyroid function are consistent with chronic renal failure.
- Systemic blood pressure measurement – indirect assessment with a Doppler sphygmomanometer (ultrasonic detection device) reveals a systolic blood pressure of 220 mmHg (upper limit for systolic blood pressure in the cat is 160–170 mmHg).

Diagnosis

Based on the information available, a diagnosis of systemic hypertension is made. The ocular manifestations are hyphaema and hypertensive retinopathy in the right eye, and glaucoma secondary to intraocular haemorrhage in the left eye.

Treatment

The preferred first-line treatment for feline systemic hypertension is amlodipine besylate (a calcium channel blocker) at a dose of 0.625–1.25 mg *per os* q24 hours. The aim of treatment is to lower the systolic blood pressure to a safe range, i.e. ≤160–170 mmHg. Some cats need more frequent dosing (amlodipine besylate q12 hours) and others require the addition of benazepril to become normotensive. Adverse effects of amlodipine besylate are uncommon but include azotaemia, lethargy, hypokalaemia, reflex tachycardia and weight loss.

   Symptomatic treatment for hyphaema can be considered with topical corticosteroid therapy, e.g. 1% prednisolone acetate q8–12 hours. Enucleation of the left eye in this cat is indicated because of pain, irreversible blindness and to prevent complications arising from progressive corneal disease.

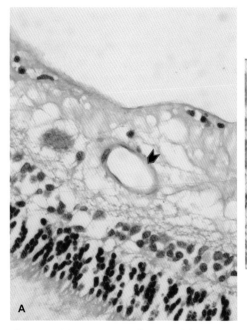
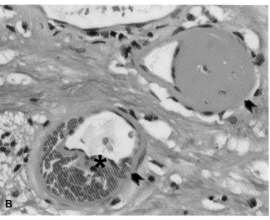

Fig. 1.1g (A) H&E section of a normal feline retina demonstrating a normal retinal arteriole (arrow) (×200). (B) H&E section of the detached retina in this hypertensive cat demonstrating two abnormal retinal arterioles (arrows) (×400). The arteriolar walls are diffusely expanded by a bright pink homogenous matrix. This is referred to as hyalinisation and results from the leakage of plasma products into the vessel wall secondary to endothelial damage. Note the haemorrhage dissecting the vessel wall (asterix) and the perivascular haemorrhage. Thickening of the vessel walls has resulted in extreme narrowing of the blood vessel lumens which are now barely visible; this degree of narrowing could result in ischaemic injury. The histopathological diagnosis is retinal and choroidal hyalinising arteriolosclerosis with intraocular haemorrhage characteristic of hypertensive retinopathy. Reproduced with permission from EJ Scurrell.

A transconjunctival procedure is performed. In addition to the clinical findings, ocular histopathology reveals retinal detachment and confirms the clinical diagnosis of glaucoma secondary to extensive intraocular haemorrhage caused by the systemic hypertension (Fig. 1.1g).

Repeated thorough physical and ophthalmic examinations as well as blood pressure measurements are recommended, e.g. every 3–6 months.

> All enucleated globes should be submitted for ocular histopathology. For routine diagnostic purposes, fixation of the globe in 10% formalin is generally appropriate, although confirmation with the chosen laboratory is recommended. Prior to fixation, as much excess extraocular tissue as possible should be removed, and the optic nerve should be left as long as possible.

Prognosis

The prognosis is good for retinal detachment secondary to systemic hypertension in that most retinas reattach if antihypertensive therapy is successful at lowering the blood pressure sufficiently. The prognosis for vision is variable because it depends on the extent and duration of retinal detachment prior to treatment, as well as the severity of any associated haemorrhage. There is evidence to suggest that the feline retina begins to degenerate within the first week of detachment. However, most cats only present when they are severely visually impaired or blind, by which stage both eyes are affected. The retinal pathology is often chronic in the eye that is affected first but is only noted when the fellow eye develops significant disease. Even if vision is not restored, continued treatment of the systemic hypertension is imperative to minimise progressive disease of other target organs (brain, heart, kidney).

Discussion

Systemic hypertension is a relatively common disease in cats older than 10 years and is usually associated with chronic renal failure, and less frequently, with hyperthyroidism and Conn's syndrome. As the eye is a target organ for hypertensive damage, the most common reason for presentation is acute blindness secondary to retinal detachment. Neurological deficits may be present and are generally the result of cerebrovascular disease. Prolonged hypertension initially leads to arteriolar vasoconstriction, manifested as narrowing and increased tortuosity of the retinal arterioles, and finally to compromise of the vascular integrity. This in turn leads to intraocular haemorrhage as well as retinal oedema and an accumulation of serous fluid which separates the neurosensory retina from the underlying retinal pigment epithelium. The ocular changes progress over several months and early diagnosis of 'at risk' cats is important in preventing blindness. Ideally any geriatric cat should have an annual blood pressure assessment together with a complete ocular examination including fundic examination. Cats with e.g. renal disease or hyperthyroidism should be monitored particularly closely.

Further reading

See Appendix 2.

History

A 9-month-old male Labrador Retriever is presented because both eyes have looked different for several months. There has been no evidence of ocular discomfort and the dog catches balls well. The dog has received his primary vaccination course and routine anthelmintic treatment and is reported to be clinically well.

Questions

1. Describe the abnormalities and pertinent normal features in Figs. 1.2a and b.
2. What differential diagnoses should be considered for this presentation?
3. What tests could you perform to make the diagnosis?

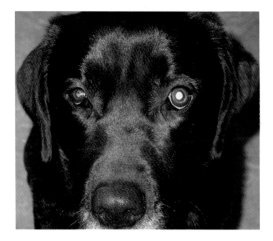

Fig. 1.2a

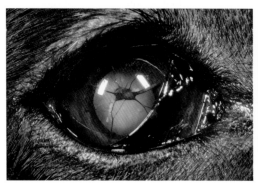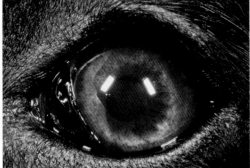

Fig. 1.2b Right eye has received a topical mydriatic agent (tropicamide).

Answers

1. What the figures show
Fig. 1.2a Left eye – is normal and shows an iris colour variation consisting of a mid brown outer zone and a dark brown pupillary zone. Right eye – has a small palpebral fissure; there is protrusion of the TEL. The pupil is small which creates a subtle anisocoria (OD < OS). The iris is slightly dark compared to the left eye. A tapetal reflection is not visible.

Fig 1.2b Both eyes are shown – the right pupil has been artificially dilated with tropicamide. Right eye – there is a structure which comprises multiple strands of iris tissue. The strands originate from the iris collarette and join at a single focal point. A cataract is present, resulting in leukocoria (white pupil).

2. Differential diagnoses
Given the history and appearance of the right eye, the following conditions should be considered:
- **Microphthalmos** This is a congenital anomaly in which the eye is abnormally small and deeply set within the orbit and has a range of concurrent defects including persistent pupillary membrane (PPM) remnants, cataract, retinal dysplasia, staphyloma, and nystagmus.
- **Nanophthalmos** A congenital anomaly in which the eye is abnormally small but otherwise normal.
- **Phthisis bulbi** Acquired end-stage atrophy of the eye following severe inflammation, ocular trauma or glaucoma. Typical features include an absence of visible signs of inflammation, an opaque cornea which prevents intraocular examination and marked hypotony (Fig. 1.2c).
- **Enophthalmos** An eye that is recessed in the orbit, causes of which include:
  - **Pain** Stimulation of the ophthalmic branch of the trigeminal nerve results in globe retraction by the retractor bulbi muscle which leads to enophthalmos and passive TEL protrusion. Conditions such as entropion and corneal ulceration often cause enophthalmos secondary to ocular surface pain. Ocular surface pain is also manifested by blepharospasm and increased lacrimation (*Ch. 5*).
  - **Horner's syndrome** Interruption of the sympathetic innervation of the eye, eyelids and orbital smooth muscle resulting in miosis, anisocoria, ptosis, narrow palpebral fissure, enophthalmos, and TEL protrusion (*Ch. 10, case 1*).
  - **Reduced volume of orbital tissue** This can arise because of dehydration, weight loss (reduction in orbital fat) or fibrosis of orbital tissues following orbital inflammation or surgery.

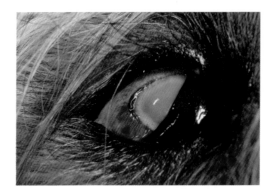

Fig. 1.2c Phthisis bulbi secondary to chronic uveitis in the right eye of a Tibetan Terrier. Note the third eyelid protrusion, increased scleral show, absence of external signs of inflammation, and diffuse corneal fibrosis.

3. Appropriate diagnostic tests

- Ocular reflexes
  - ◦ Pupillary light reflex – positive direct and consensual OU
  - ◦ Dazzle reflex – positive OU
- Menace response – positive OS, negative OD

In this dog, these results are consistent with absent vision but some retinal and optic nerve function in the right eye.

- Examination with a focal light source – in the right eye, slit-lamp biomicroscopy shows that the structure originating at the iris collarette converges at a focal point on the anterior lens capsule, consistent with a PPM.
- Tonometry – IOP 15 mmHg OU
- B-mode ocular ultrasound – this is indicated to evaluate the posterior segment when the anterior segment is opaque, and to take measurements. Axial globe length is the distance between the centre of the cornea and the posterior pole. Axial lens length is the distance between the centre of the anterior and posterior lens capsules.

    The ultrasound reveals an axial globe length of 20.8 mm OS (within normal limits) and 18.5 mm OD, which confirms microphthalmos in the right eye (Fig. 1.2d). The right lens is hyperechoic and slightly smaller than the left lens (axial length 7.1 mm compared to 7.3 mm, both within normal limits); the hyperechogenicity is consistent with a cataract.

There is no change in the appearance or apparent comfort level of the right eye following the application of topical anaesthetic eye drops, which rules out enophthalmos because of ocular surface pain. The position of the TEL in the right eye does not change following the application of topical 1% phenylephrine, which makes Horner's syndrome an unlikely cause of the TEL protrusion (*Ch. 10, case 1*). The remainder of the ophthalmic examination reveals no additional abnormalities and a general physical examination is unremarkable.

> A single drop of a topical anaesthetic will anaesthetise the ocular surface (conjunctiva and cornea) within approximately 10 s. Anaesthesia lasts for about 45 min in the normal dog eye (25 min in the cat). The depth and duration of anaesthesia can be increased by the repeat application of the topical anaesthetic, e.g. one drop applied twice over one minute. The application of a topical anaesthetic can be a simple way of differentiating surface ocular pain from pain caused by intraocular or orbital disease.

Diagnosis

Based on the information available, a diagnosis of microphthalmos in the right eye is made.

Treatment

No treatment is indicated for the majority of eyes affected with microphthalmos. In a small number of dogs, recurrent conjunctivitis may develop because of poor tear drainage and/or entropion because of poor eyelid-to-globe apposition. Conjunctivitis is usually managed conservatively with topical lubricant and antibiotic therapy; entropion should be surgically corrected. Congenital cataract associated with microphthalmos is typically non-progressive, and cataract removal in a

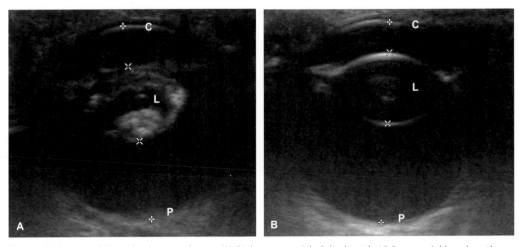

Fig.1.2d Horizontal B-mode ultrasound scan. (A) Right eye – axial globe length 18.5 mm, axial lens length 7.1 mm; hyperechoic lens. This is consistent with microphthalmos and cataract. (B) Left eye – axial globe length 20.8 mm, axial lens length 7.3 mm. C, cornea; L, lens; P, posterior limit of globe; 'x' and '+' represent points of measurement for the axial length of lens and globe respectively.

microphthalmic eye is associated with an increased risk of complications. Cataract removal is not considered in this dog because vision in the left eye is considered to be normal.

Prognosis
Most microphthalmic eyes remain stable as the associated ocular abnormalities are typically non-progressive. The prognosis for the right eye is therefore considered to be good.

Discussion
Microphthalmos is described in many species and in many different dog breeds. Although typically unilateral it may be bilateral but not necessarily symmetrical. Abnormalities range from mild to severe and vision may be normal, reduced or absent. In addition, microphthalmic eyes commonly have clinically insignificant iris hypoplasia seen as miosis (because of hypoplasia of the iris dilator muscle) and a darkened iris, as in this dog. Miosis and darkening of the iris can also occur with anterior uveitis and should be ruled out on the basis of other clinical signs (*Ch. 7, case 1, Fig. 7.1e*). Although the cause of microphthalmos is often unknown, a heritable basis is described in several dog breeds including the Dobermann Pinscher, Miniature Schnauzer, English Cocker Spaniel and the Australian Shepherd. Animals with reduced pigment (melanin) in the body (subalbinism) are also commonly affected, e.g. merle collies. Regardless of the severity of the defect, affected animals should not be used for breeding.

Further reading
See Appendix 2.

History

A 5-year-old male neutered Weimaraner is presented with a two-day history of a prominent red eye, reduced appetite and lethargy. The dog has received routine vaccinations and anthelmintic treatment.

Questions

1. Describe the abnormalities and pertinent normal features in Figs. 1.3a and b.
2. What differential diagnoses should be considered for this presentation?
3. What tests could you perform to make the diagnosis?

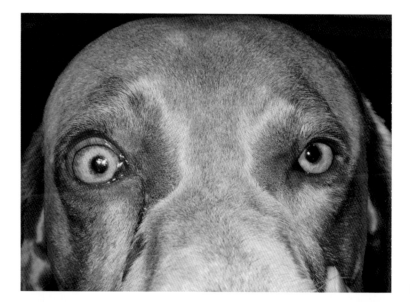

Fig. 1.3a

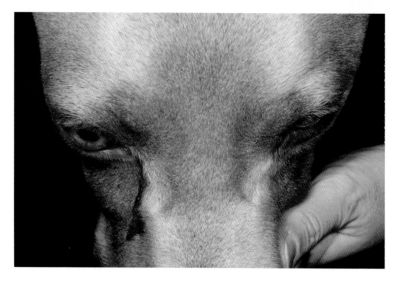

Fig. 1.3b

Answers

1. What the figures show

Fig. 1.3a Both eyes are shown, the left eye is normal. Right eye – there is marked periocular swelling, erythema of the upper and lower eyelid skin and a widened palpebral fissure (OD > OS). The Purkinje images are disrupted and displaced. There is epiphora, TEL protrusion and hyperaemia of the bulbar conjunctiva.

Fig. 1.3b Aerial view of both eyes. Right eye – there is an obvious anterior displacement of the eye; this appears as a larger visible surface area of cornea when compared to the left eye. The periocular swelling ventral to the eye is more evident with this view.

2. Differential diagnoses

Given the appearance of the right eye, the clinical diagnosis is exophthalmos. The following conditions should be considered:

- **Orbital neoplasia** This can be primary (60–70% of tumours) or secondary, arising from adjacent structures or metastasis from distant sites. Orbital neoplasia is more likely in older dogs (mean age 9.5 years) and is characterised by a slowly progressive unilateral exophthalmos with variable degrees of strabismus. Affected dogs are typically but not exclusively non-painful. Indentation of the caudal globe can be seen on fundic examination and with some imaging modalities (ultrasonography, MRI and CT).
- **Orbital cellulitis/abscess** This is most common in young dogs (mean age 4 years) and is characterised by acute onset unilateral exophthalmos, and pain on opening the mouth and palpation of the globe and periocular region. Associated clinical signs include an ipsilateral swelling of the oral mucosa caudal to the last upper premolar, pyrexia, anorexia and neutrophilia. The cause of the cellulitis/abscess is not always identified but includes an orbital foreign body, dental problem or from haematogenous spread.
- **Myositis**
  - **Extraocular polymyositis (EOM)** Inflammation of the extraocular muscles causes bilateral but not necessarily symmetrical ocular signs including exophthalmos, strabismus and impaired globe movement. EOM has been described in several breeds but is most commonly seen in the Golden Retriever (*case 4, this chapter*).
  - **Masticatory/eosinophilic myositis** Acute inflammation of the masticatory muscles (masseter, temporal, pterygoid and digastric muscles) causes anorexia, pyrexia, and bilateral exophthalmos. Chronic disease results in fibrosis of the masticatory muscles and can lead to enophthalmos, entropion, TEL protrusion, and impaired vision.
- **Trauma**
  - **Orbital haematoma** This occurs most commonly following proptosis as a result of severe trauma, e.g. road traffic accident, and is often associated with subconjunctival haemorrhage and lagophthalmos.
  - **Orbital emphysema** This can arise as a complication of enucleation, especially in brachycephalic breeds, as well as from fractures involving the frontal sinus.
  - **Proptosis** This term describes the sudden forward displacement of the eye with subsequent entrapment behind the eyelids (*Ch. 12, case 1*).
  - **Orbital fractures** Fractures of the frontal, temporal and zygomatic bone can result in exophthalmos or enophthalmos, strabismus, orbital and periocular haemorrhage, pain, and facial asymmetry.
- **Abnormalities of the zygomatic salivary gland** Neoplasia, inflammation of the zygomatic salivary gland (sialoadenitis) or leakage of saliva can cause exophthalmos. There is often a history

of trauma with the non-neoplastic conditions. Oral examination may reveal distension of the zygomatic papilla.
- **Vascular anomalies** Orbital varices and arteriovenous fistulas are rare congenital anomalies that may cause pulsating or intermittent exophthalmos.

3. Appropriate diagnostic tests
- Ocular reflexes
  - Pupillary light reflex – positive direct and consensual OS, negative direct and consensual OD
  - Dazzle reflex – positive OS, negative OD
  - Palpebral reflex – positive OU but reduced OD
  - Vestibulo-ocular reflex – positive OU but reduced OD
- Menace response – positive OS, equivocal OD

In this dog, these results are consistent with blindness, absent retinal and optic nerve function, reduced ocular motility and lagophthalmos in the right eye.

- Ophthalmoscopy – this reveals an extensive area of hyporeflectivity in the tapetal fundus in the right eye, and no abnormalities in the left eye.
- Fluorescein dye
  - Staining – negative OS, positive diffuse stippling of the axial cornea OD. This is indicative of suboptimal ocular surface health in the right eye, most likely because of the lagophthalmos.
  - Jones test (fluorescein dye passage test) – positive OS, negative OD. This is consistent with reduced tear drainage on the right side because of compression of the nasolacrimal punctum by anterior displacement of the globe.
- Tonometry – IOP 18 mmHg OS, 27 mmHg OD. In the absence of other signs of glaucoma (e.g. mydriasis), the elevated IOP in the right eye is consistent with increased intraorbital pressure causing ocular hypertension rather than glaucoma.
- Luedde or Hertel exophthalmometer – an instrument specifically designed to measure the distance between the cornea and the lateral orbital ligament. It is not routinely used in veterinary ophthalmology. Examination from an aerial perspective confirms that the right eye is displaced anteriorly (Fig. 1.3b).

On further examination there is pain and increased resistance to retropulsion of the right eye; retropulsion of the left eye is normal. There is pain when the mouth is opened but no intraoral abnormalities are observed. A general physical examination is otherwise unremarkable except for mild bilateral mandibular lymphadenopathy.

Further diagnostic tests
- Laboratory tests – routine haematology, biochemistry and urine analysis are unremarkable
- Imaging
  - B-mode ocular and orbital ultrasound – this is indicated to evaluate the retrobulbar space and the orbit. It reveals a hypoechoic oval mass with a hyperechoic rim within the retrobulbar space of the right eye. The mass is causing marked indentation of the posterior aspect of the globe which is consistent with the fundoscopic findings (Fig. 1.3c).
  - Abdominal ultrasonography – unremarkable
  - Thoracic radiography – unremarkable
  - MRI – this is performed to evaluate the full extent of the orbital lesion and to determine if surgical management is possible. The dorsal T1 image confirms the presence of the retrobulbar mass identified on the ultrasound examination. The mass is isointense to brain tissue, has a hypointense core, and indents the posterior aspect of the globe (Fig. 1.3d).

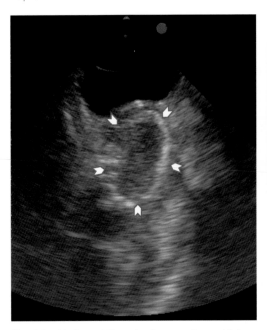

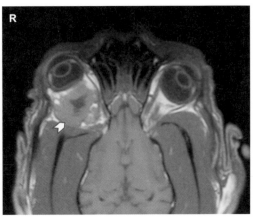

Fig. 1.3d MRI scan (dorsal T1 image). A large retrobulbar mass (arrow) indents the posterior aspect of the eye. Reproduced with permission from R Dennis, Animal Heath Trust.

Fig. 1.3c Horizontal B-mode ultrasound scan (right eye). A hypoechoic oval mass (arrows) within the retrobulbar space indents the posterior aspect of the eye.

- Fine-needle aspiration (FNA) for bacteriology and cytology – under general anaesthesia and with ultrasound guidance, an FNA of the retrobulbar mass (via an intraoral approach) and the right mandibular lymph node is performed. Cytological examination reveals a monomorphic population of large neoplastic lymphocytes in both the orbit and lymph node (Fig. 1.3e). There is no growth on bacterial culture.

> There is a close association between the soft tissue floor of the orbit, and the maxilla and the mandible. With some orbital disorders, opening of the mouth can result in discomfort because the coronoid process of the ramus of the mandible presses on the soft tissue floor of the orbit. Careful inspection of the oral mucosa caudal to the last upper premolar on the affected side (conscious or under general anaesthesia) to look for abnormalities such as redness or swelling is important in the evaluation of suspected orbital conditions.

Diagnosis

Based on the information available, a diagnosis of orbital lymphoma on the right side is made.

Treatment

The treatment of exophthalmos depends on the underlying cause. Clinical staging is indicated in cases of lymphoma and typically includes a complete blood count, biochemistry, urinalysis, diagnostic imaging (abdominal and thoracic), and, if indicated, bone marrow evaluation and immunophenotyping. The reader is referred to appropriate sources for further information.

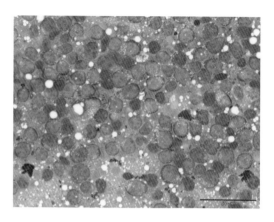

Fig. 1.3e Orbital FNA depicting neoplastic lymphocytes. Wright's Giemsa stain. Bar = 50 μm. Reproduced with permission from EJ Scurrell.

Non-specific therapy for exophthalmos includes a topical lubricant to minimise the risk of corneal ulceration because of exposure. Many topical lubricants are commercially available – a paraffin-based, bland ophthalmic ointment applied generously q4–6 hours is appropriate. Placement of a temporary tarsorrhaphy (eyelid sutures that partially or completely close the palpebral fissure) is an alternative means of protecting the ocular surface until the exophthalmos improves or resolves. This can be performed whilst the animal is under general anaesthesia for imaging.

Prognosis

In this dog the prognosis for the rapid resolution of the exophthalmos is good if there is a satisfactory response to chemotherapy. The exophthalmos should improve within several days and/or resolve during the first 1–2 weeks of treatment. However, prolonged or severe exophthalmos can result in corneal ulceration and blindness because of optic nerve damage.

Most preferred chemotherapy protocols will result in an 80–90% rate of clinical remission, with median survival times of 12 months. Approximately 25% of affected dogs survive longer than two years.

Discussion

Most orbital space-occupying lesions are neoplastic in the dog. Orbital neoplasia usually causes a slowly progressive, non-painful exophthalmos, in contrast to the acute onset, painful exophthalmos typical of an inflammatory process. However, orbital lymphoma can mimic inflammation because it often has an acute onset and can be painful. Diagnostic imaging is always indicated for a thorough evaluation of exophthalmos. Orbital ultrasound is relatively simple and inexpensive to perform but the interpretation of orbital scans is often challenging, even for an experienced ultrasonographer. Plain skull radiography is only helpful if there is bony involvement. MRI and CT can provide further information about the nature and extent of the orbital lesion which can then facilitate accurate planning of orbital surgery (if indicated).

Further reading
See Appendix 2.

History

A 1-year-old female Miniature Shorthaired Dachsund is presented with a five-day history of 'bulging eyes'. The dog has received routine vaccinations and regular anthelmintic treatment, and is reported to be otherwise clinically well.

Questions

1. Describe the abnormalities and pertinent normal features in Fig. 1.4a.
2. What differential diagnoses should be considered for this presentation?
3. What tests could you perform to make the diagnosis?

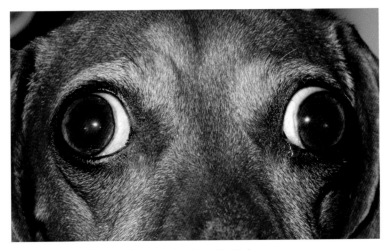

Fig. 1.4a Reproduced with permission from EA Giuliano.

Answers

1. What the figure shows
Fig. 1.4a The left and right eyes are similar except for the presence of a scant mucoid discharge in the left eye. There is a startled expression and symmetrical exotropia, i.e. a divergent strabismus or lateral deviation. Evidence of exotropia includes an increase in the amount of visible sclera on the medial aspect of the globe and the abnormal position of the Purkinje images (see Fig. 1.4b for comparison). The exotropia has resulted in misalignment between the camera flash and the visual axis and as a result a tapetal reflection is not visible. There is a mild exophthalmos with associated widening of the palpebral fissure and exposure of the sclera on the dorsal and ventral aspects of the eye. The TEL is in a normal position. The pupil size is appropriate for the ambient lighting.

2. Differential diagnoses
Given the history and the appearance of both eyes, the following conditions should be considered:
- **EOM** An acute inflammatory process confined to the extraocular muscles (excluding the retractor bulbi). EOM is characterised by bilateral exophthalmos and strabismus and a classic startled expression; TEL protrusion, pain and visible signs of inflammation are absent. Although there is an idiopathic predisposition for the young female Golden Retriever, EOM has been described in many dog breeds.
- **Masticatory muscle myositis (MMM)** An acute inflammatory process involving the muscles of mastication (masseter, temporal, pterygoid and digastric muscles). MMM is characterised by bilateral exophthalmos, TEL protrusion and congestion of the conjunctival and episcleral vessels. Concurrent non-ocular signs are more often the reason for presentation and include lethargy, pyrexia, and anorexia, the latter primarily because of jaw pain. Jaw pain results from pressure applied by the ramus of the mandible on the swollen soft tissue floor of the orbit when the mouth is opened. The masticatory muscles are often visibly swollen and painful when palpated. Haematological and biochemical abnormalities include a leukocytosis, eosinophilia and elevated creatinine phosphokinase. The masticatory muscles are composed of unique type 2M myofibre, for which specific autoantibodies can be identified. The serum 2M antibody test and immunocytochemical staining on muscle tissue are important diagnostic tests for MMM. Chronic or severe disease leads to fibrosis of the muscles and subsequent enophthalmos, entropion, TEL protrusion, impaired vision and trismus.
- **Physiological exotropia and exophthalmos** The optical axes are offset by approximately 20° in a rostrolateral direction in the normal dog, resulting in good binocular vision and dorsomedial positioning of the Purkinje images. The position of the optical axes and the depth of the orbit depends on skull shape – brachycephalic breeds have a tendency for mild bilateral exotropia and exophthalmos that is within normal limits for the breed type (Fig. 1.4b).
- **Orbital lymphoma** Lymphoma can present as acute onset, unilateral or bilateral orbital disease – the clinical signs mimic an inflammatory rather than a neoplastic process. With the exception of lymphoma, orbital neoplasia is more typically unilateral, non-painful and slowly progressive in nature (*case 3, this chapter*).
- **Abnormalities of the zygomatic salivary gland** Neoplasia, inflammation of the zygomatic salivary gland (sialoadenitis) or leakage of saliva can cause exophthalmos. There is often a history of trauma with the non-neoplastic conditions. Oral examination may reveal distension of the zygomatic papilla.

3. Appropriate diagnostic tests
- Ocular reflexes

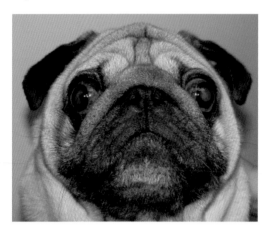

Fig. 1.4b Bilateral breed-related exotropia, exophthalmos and macropalpebral fissure in an adult Pug. Reproduced with permission from DJ Gould.

- ○ Pupillary light reflex – direct and consensual positive OU
- ○ Dazzle reflex – positive OU
- ○ Palpebral reflex – positive OU
- ○ Vestibulo-ocular reflex – positive but reduced OU
- Vision assessment
  - ○ Menace response – positive OU
  - ○ Visual placing and tracking reflexes – positive OU

In this dog, these results are consistent with reduced ocular motility in both eyes.

- Tonometry – IOP 26 mmHg OU. In the absence of signs of glaucoma (e.g. mydriasis, corneal oedema, episcleral congestion, pain), the mildly elevated IOP is consistent with increased intraorbital pressure causing ocular hypertension.

There is mild resistance to retropulsion of both eyes but no obvious pain. The remainder of the ophthalmic examination reveals no additional abnormalities and a general physical examination is unremarkable.

Further diagnostic tests

- Forced duction test – this test helps to differentiate mechanical restriction from a neurological disorder in an eye with reduced motility. It can be performed in a conscious (active forced duction) or unconscious, anaesthetised animal (passive forced duction).

  A passive forced duction test is performed in this dog. Each eye in turn is grasped with fine rat-toothed forceps close to the limbus and is moved only partially in all directions. This is a positive result which excludes a neurological problem and suggests that the reduced vestibulo-ocular reflex is the result of a restrictive (mechanical) problem.
- Laboratory tests – routine haematology, biochemistry and urine analysis are recommended prior to starting treatment; the results are unremarkable.
- B-mode ocular ultrasound – this reveals thickening of the extraocular muscles in both eyes, and associated enlargement of the retrobulbar cone (Fig. 1.4c).
- Orbital MRI – this confirms marked thickening of the extraocular muscles and reveals contrast enhancement consistent with inflammation (Fig. 1.4d).

Diagnosis

Based on the information available, a diagnosis of bilateral extraocular polymyositis is made.

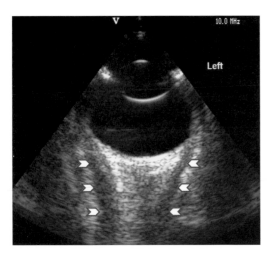

Fig. 1.4c Horizontal B-mode ultrasound scan. Marked thickening of the extraocular muscles of the left eye (arrows). Reproduced with permission from R Dennis, Animal Health Trust.

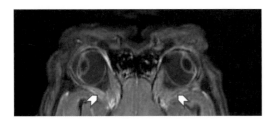

Fig. 1.4d MRI image (dorsal T1 post contrast). Marked thickening and enhancement of the extraocular muscles of both eyes (arrows). Reproduced with permission from R Dennis, Animal Health Trust.

Treatment

The mainstay of treatment for EOM is systemic corticosteroid therapy at immunosuppressive doses. Prednisolone, 1.1 mg/kg q12 hours for three weeks, is recommended (Ramsey *et al.*, 1995). The prednisolone can then be tapered over several weeks. Adjunctive therapy with azathioprine may need to be considered in patients that cannot tolerate the side-effects of corticosteroid therapy or become refractory to prednisolone therapy alone. Alternative immunomodulatory therapy with oral cyclophosphamide alone, and a combination of oxytetracycline and niacinamide have also been reported for this condition.

Prognosis

With early accurate diagnosis and appropriate treatment, the prognosis for EOM is generally good and clinical signs usually resolve. However, recurrence is common and is reported to be as high as 80%, with 10% of dogs experiencing multiple recurrences (Ramsey *et al.*, 1995). Recurrence was found to be most likely if the initial dose of prednisolone was reduced before the end of the recommended three-week period. A small number of dogs require low-dose, long-term therapy to maintain remission.

Discussion

EOM is an idiopathic inflammatory condition that probably has an immune-mediated component; this assumption is based on the pattern of muscle involvement, histopathological features and response to treatment. A common history of a non-specific stressor (e.g. a stay in boarding kennels, surgery, oestrus) prior to the onset of clinical signs has been noted in some cases.

The startled facial expression is virtually pathognomic for EOM and the diagnosis can usually be made from the characteristic clinical appearance alone. In addition to the clinical signs described above, less common clinical signs include conjunctival hyperaemia, chemosis, fundic changes and visual impairment. The lack of TEL protrusion in this condition is especially noteworthy as this is in contrast to most orbital disease in dogs (*case 3, this chapter*). Advanced imaging in the form of ocular and orbital ultrasonography, CT and MRI helps localise the abnormality and confirm the diagnosis. Ultrasonography, although quick and relatively inexpensive to perform, does not necessarily provide precise information about the nature of the problem and the tissues involved. Although MMM can also cause bilateral exophthalmos, the clinical presentation is very different to that for EOM (see earlier). The clinical differences between these two myopathies arise from the fact that the muscle groups have different embryological origins. The type 2M myofibre is unique to the masticatory muscles and can be identified with serology (2M autoantibodies) and immunocytochemistry on frozen muscle sections; the masticatory muscles are easy to biopsy as they are large and readily accessible (Melmed *et al.*, 2004). Although the extraocular muscles can be biopsied, the procedure is challenging and is generally unnecessary as histopathology of the muscles is non-specific (myonecrosis with a mononuclear infiltrate) and type 2M fibres are not present. Serology and muscle biopsy are therefore useful diagnostic tests to confirm the diagnosis of MMM but are not indicated for EOM.

References and further reading

Melmed C, Shelton GD, Bergman R, Barton C. (2004) Masticatory muscle myositis: pathogenesis, diagnosis and treatment. *Compend Contin Ed.*, 590–605.

Ramsey DT, Hamor RE, Gerding PA, Knight B. Clinical and immunohistochemical characteristics of bilateral extraocular polymyositis of dogs. *Proc Am Coll Vet Ophthalmol*, 1995; 130–132.

Williams DL (2008) Extraocular myositis in dogs. *Vet Clin North Am: Small Animal Pract*, 38, 347–59.

See Appendix 2.

CHAPTER 2

Eyelid Abnormalities

Introduction

The eyelid is a mucocutaneous junction, and as such provides an interface between the skin and the ocular surface. It has an important role in ocular surface health because of its contribution to the mucin layer of the precorneal tear film from the meibomian glands. Eyelid abnormalities are very common in the dog, less so in the cat. They generally go unnoticed unless they cause an ocular discharge or ocular discomfort.

Small Animal Ophthalmology: What's Your Diagnosis? First Edition. Heidi Featherstone, Elaine Holt.
© 2011 by Heidi Featherstone and Elaine Holt. Published 2011 by Blackwell Publishing Ltd.

A one-year-old male Weimaraner is presented with a two-month history of painful and watery eyes. The dog has received routine vaccinations and regular anthelmintic treatment, and is otherwise clinically well.

Questions

1. Describe the abnormalities in the eyes in Figs. 2.1a, b, and c.
2. What differential diagnoses should be considered for this presentation?
3. What tests could you perform to make the diagnosis?

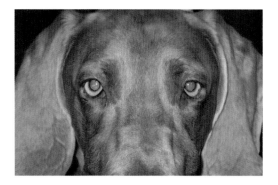

Fig. 2.1a

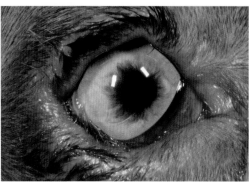

Fig. 2.1b

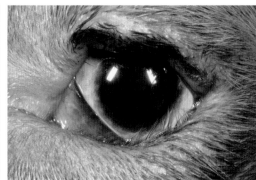

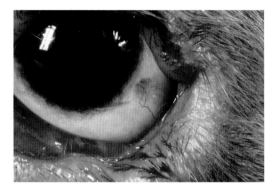

Fig. 2.1c

Answers

1. What the figures show
Fig. 2.1a Both eyes – there is mild epiphora, third eyelid protrusion and conjunctival hyperaemia. The hairs on the lower eyelid are wet and the eyelid skin is erythematous.

Fig. 2.1b Both eyes – there is marked inversion of the lower eyelid margin and resulting trichiasis. The contour of the upper eyelid is irregular or 'notched' and there are several fine distichia. There is relative anisocoria (OD < OS) because of different ambient room light. The Purkinje images are normal.

Fig. 2.1c Left eye – there is localised superficial keratitis which appears as corneal vascularisation within the ventrolateral quadrant.

> The 'notched' appearance in the upper eyelid is a common feature in some dog breeds. The facial nerve innervates the levator anguli oculi medialis muscle in the medial region, and the oculomotor nerve innervates the levator palpebrae superioris muscle in the central region. The position of the 'notch' represents the junction between these two regions.

> Approximately four days after corneal injury blood vessels begin to grow at the limbus and progress at an average rate of 1 mm per day. This fact is helpful when trying to determine how long corneal disease has been present.

2. Differential diagnoses
Given the history of ocular discomfort and the appearance of both eyes, the following conditions should be considered:

- **Entropion** The inversion or inward turning of all or part of the eyelid margin. The resulting trichiasis causes discomfort, conjunctivitis, keratitis and sometimes corneal ulceration. Entropion can involve any part of the eyelid but lower lateral entropion is most frequently encountered in clinical practice.
- **Eyelid agenesis or coloboma** Localised absence of eyelid tissue results in increased exposure of the ocular surface, trichiasis and a reduced ability to blink; together these cause conjunctivitis and keratitis, with associated discomfort. Eyelid agenesis is most common in the lateral upper eyelid of cats; it is rarely seen in the dog.
- **Distichiasis** This is a common condition in which extra eyelashes arise from the region of the meibomian glands and emerge out of, or just posterior to, the gland openings along the eyelid margin (*Ch. 5, case 1, Diagram 5.1*). Distichiasis tends to occur in dogs less than one year old. It is often an incidental finding, but it can cause increased lacrimation, epiphora, and blepharospasm; corneal ulceration is uncommon. Predisposed breeds are the Cocker Spaniel (American and English), Boxer, English Bulldog, Flat-Coated Retriever, Shih Tzu, Pekingese, Poodle, Dachsund and Jack Russell Terrier (*case 2, this chapter*).
- **Ectopic cilia** This is a condition in which extra eyelashes arise from the region of the meibomian glands but, in contrast to distichiasis, emerge through the palpebral conjunctiva 4–6 mm from the eyelid margin. Ectopic cilia most commonly occur in the centre of the upper eyelid and cause direct irritation to the ocular surface (*Ch. 5, case 1, Diagram 5.1*). The typical clinical presentation

is acute onset blepharospasm, lacrimation and corneal ulceration in a young dog (usually less than one year old). Clinical signs may be intermittent because ectopic cilia eventually fall out, only to regrow several weeks later. Predisposed breeds include the Lhasa Apso, Pekingese, Shih Tzu, Poodle, English Bulldog, Flat-Coated Retriever and Boxer (*Ch. 5, case 1*).

- **Trichiasis** This is a condition in which periocular hairs growing in a normal location are abnormally directed towards the ocular surface. If severe, trichiasis can cause conjunctivitis and keratitis, with associated discomfort. Trichiasis results from entropion and eyelid agenesis and can also be associated with the nasal folds, medial canthus and caruncle.
- **Corneal ulceration** Pain accompanies corneal ulceration. Superficial ulcers are usually more painful than deep ulcers, because the anterior corneal stroma has a high proportion of pain receptors, whereas the deep corneal stroma is rich in pressure receptors.
- **Tear film disorders** Both quantitative (keratoconjunctivitis sicca) and qualititative tear film disorders can cause ocular discomfort, mucoid discharge, conjunctivitis and keratitis (*Ch. 4, case 3*).

3. Appropriate diagnostic tests
- Ocular reflexes
  - Pupillary light reflex – direct and consensual positive OU
  - Dazzle reflex – positive OU
  - Palpebral reflex – positive OU
- Menace response – positive OU
- Examination with a focal light source – in both eyes, the entire length of the lower eyelid turns inwards and manual eversion of the skin is necessary to observe the eyelid margin. The lower eyelid margin is lighter in colour than the upper; this is consistent with temporary depigmentation because of persistent contact between the eyelid margin and the moist ocular surface. The lower eyelid is everted and straightened by gentle traction in a lateral direction, revealing that the eyelid is abnormally long. There are several fine hairs along the eyelid margins in both eyes, consistent with distichiasis (*Ch. 2, case 2*).
- Schirmer tear test – this is not performed, because of the excessive lacrimation in both eyes.
- Fluorescein dye – negative staining OU
- Tonometry – IOP 18 mmHg OU

The blepharospasm resolves in both eyes following administration of a topical anaesthetic drug. The remainder of the ophthalmic examination reveals no additional abnormalities and a general physical examination is unremarkable.

A single drop of a topical anaesthetic drug will anaesthetise the ocular surface (conjunctiva and cornea) within approximately 10 s. Anaesthesia lasts for about 45 min in the normal dog eye (25 min in the cat). The depth and duration of anaesthesia can be increased by the repeat application of the topical anaesthetic, e.g. one drop applied twice in one minute. The application of a topical anaesthetic can be a simple way of differentiating ocular surface pain from pain caused by intraocular or orbital disease; it can also temporarily relieve spastic entropion.

Diagnosis
Based on the information available, a diagnosis of entropion and distichiasis is made in both eyes. There is also superficial keratitis in the left eye.

The distichiasis is considered to be an incidental finding. The low number of the distichia and their soft appearance suggest that they are unlikely to be clinically significant compared to the discomfort caused by the entropion.

Treatment

Many surgical techniques have been described for the correction of entropion in the dog. The technique chosen depends on the age and breed of dog, the type of entropion, the degree of corneal involvement, whether there has been previous eyelid surgery, and surgeon preference.

Both lower eyelids are shortened and everted by a combined technique comprising a full thickness wedge resection and Hotz-Celsus procedure (Read & Broun, 2007; Diagram 2.1). Absorbable suture material (6/0 polyglactin) is used because removal of sutures close to the eye is difficult in conscious animals. A topical broad-spectrum antibiotic is administered q12 hours in both eyes for five days following surgery; systemic broad-spectrum antibiotic and NSAID therapy are prescribed for 7–10 days.

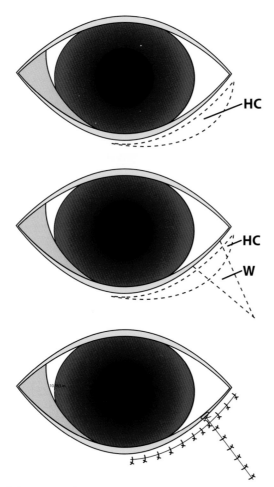

Diagram 2.1 Eversion and shortening of the eyelid by a combined Hotz-Celsus procedure and full thickness wedge resection (based on the technique described by Read & Broun, 2007). (A) Skin incisions for Hotz-Celsus procedure. (B) Skin incisions for wedge resection. The Hotz-Celsus procedure is closed with one layer of skin sutures; the wedge resection is closed in two layers (subdermis and skin). Absorbable 6/0 suture material is used. HC, Hotz-Celsus; W, wedge. Illustration by S Scurrell.

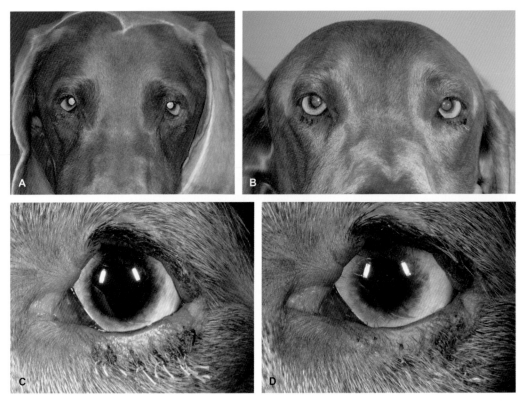

Fig. 2.1d (A) Immediate postoperative appearance. (B) Two weeks postoperatively. (C) Left eye at two weeks. The eyelid conformation is good; the skin sutures are moderately encrusted. (D) Left eye following removal of skin sutures.

The topical application of ocular medication can cause mild and transient blepharospasm. This blepharospasm can lead to a recurrence of entropion in an eye in which surgery has only recently corrected the eyelid position. For this reason the frequency of postoperative topical treatment is kept to a minimum, e.g. q12 hours.

Immediately after surgery there is mild lower ectropion in the left eye because of chemosis and eyelid swelling; this is a common and acceptable finding at this stage (Fig. 2.1d, A). Both eyes are comfortable and have good eyelid conformation two weeks after surgery (Fig. 2.1d, B). The sutures are moderately encrusted with discharge, which is also to be expected (Fig. 2.1d, C). Although the suture material is absorbable, the majority of the sutures are removed to facilitate healing and because the dog's level of co-operation is excellent (Fig. 2.1d, D). Following surgery there is no evidence of ocular irritation, which confirms that the distichiasis is clinically insignificant in this dog (*case 2, this chapter*).

Prognosis

The prognosis for resolution of the entropion is good with correct and careful case management. It is, however, important to caution the owner that repeat surgery may be necessary in some dogs.

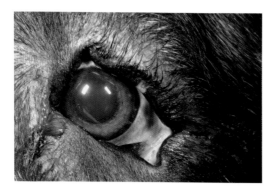

Fig. 2.1e 'Diamond eye' in the left eye of a young St Bernard dog.

Discussion

Entropion is a common condition in the dog. The pathophysiology is complex and involves the relationship between the eyelid and counterpressure from the globe, tone of the orbicularis oculi muscle and size of the palpebral fissure. Contributing factors include age, gender, skull conformation and, in some breeds, the degree of facial skin folds. Entropion can be classified as either primary (congenital and developmental), or secondary (spastic and cicatricial). Entropion causes trichiasis and, subsequently, ocular surface pain, which in turn causes increased lacrimation and enophthalmos. Enophthalmos leads to loss of support to the eyelid margin and exacerbates the entropion.

Each dog must be assessed carefully to identify the precise nature of the entropion so that the appropriate surgical technique can be selected. Trends are recognised with certain breed types: in hunting breeds (e.g. Labrador Retriever, Pointer) the lateral two thirds to three quarters of the lower eyelid is usually involved. In large and giant breeds (e.g. Great Dane, St Bernard) the palpebral fissure is excessively large, which results in central ectropion and lateral entropion – often referred to as 'diamond eye' (Fig. 2.1e). Medial lower entropion is common in toy and brachycephalic breeds (*Ch. 8, case 3*). Excessive facial skin has a strong influence on eyelid conformation in some breeds, e.g. Chow Chow, Shar Pei, and in these dogs eyelid surgery alone may not be sufficient to correct entropion. The surgical correction of entropion complicated by excessive facial folds is challenging. One surgical approach is the combination of a rhytidectomy (face-lift) followed by eyelid surgery (Fig. 2.1f A-G). It is beneficial to perform this as a two-stage procedure, so that the eyelid conformation can be reassessed following the rhytidectomy, and to ensure that the appropriate entropion technique is selected. A two-step procedure also avoids prolonged general anaesthesia.

Although surgery is indicated in most cases of canine entropion, conservative management in the form of a topical ophthalmic lubricant may be sufficient to alleviate mild discomfort. This is particularly true in young dogs with mild or intermittent entropion. This conservative approach has the advantage of allowing the skull to grow and mature, which may lead to a resolution of the entropion in a few dogs. There is no specific age at which entropion surgery should be performed – surgery is always indicated when there is ocular discomfort. Repeat surgery is most likely with complex forms of entropion, and if surgery is performed before the dog is fully mature, regardless of the breed. An important exception to this is the Shar Pei puppy, where temporary 'tacking' sutures to evert the eyelid margins, performed before 16 weeks of age, may preclude the need for permanent surgery later. If the onset of entropion occurs in a Shar Pei older than this, some form of corrective eyelid surgery is almost always indicated.

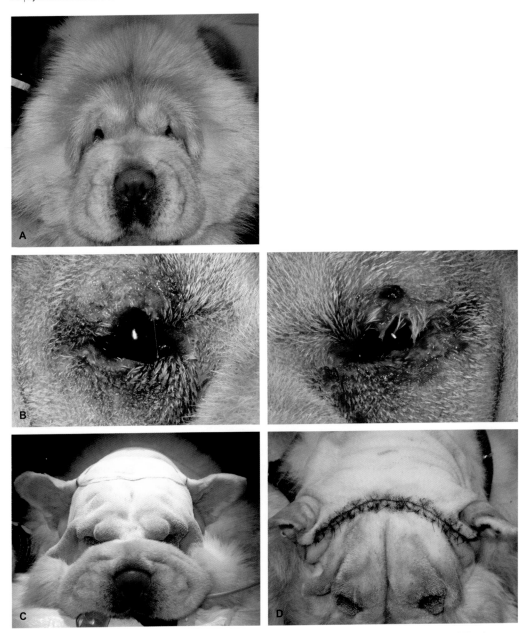

Fig. 2.1f (A) One-year-old Chow Chow with excessive facial and periocular skin, which makes it difficult to see both eyes. (B) There is bilateral mucoid discharge with a strand of mucus spanning the palpebral fissure in the right eye. In both eyes the palpebral fissure is irregular and the margin of the upper and lower eyelids is not visible; this is consistent with inversion of the eyelid margin. The ocular surface is lustrous and the Purkinje images are normal. (C) Area of skin to be excised for the rhytidectomy (dog under general anaesthesia). (D) Immediate appearance following rhytidectomy (dog under general anaesthesia). The skin wound is positioned just rostral to the ears.

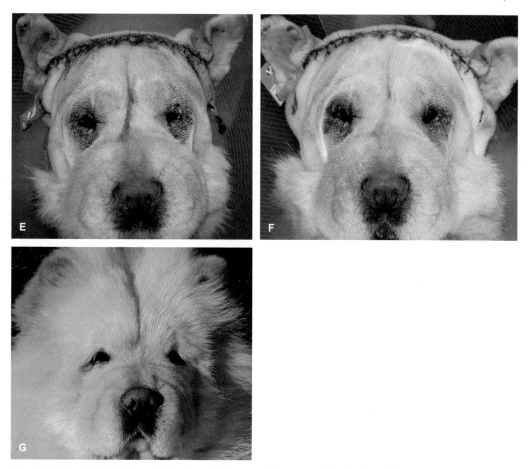

Fig. 2.1f (Cont'd) (E) 24 hours following rhytidectomy. Elevation of the forehead skin improves the eyelid conformation but lower entropion persists, especially in the left eye. The ends of Penrose drains are visible on each side of the face. (F) 24 hours following entropion surgery. Both upper and lower eyelids have been everted using a Hotz-Celsus technique. In addition, both lower eyelids have been shortened by a full thickness wedge resection. There is mild chemosis, eyelid swelling and upper ectropion; these are acceptable findings at this stage. The Penrose drains have been removed. (G) One year following rhytidectomy and entropion surgery.

References and further reading

Read RA & Broun HC (2007) Entropion correction in dogs and cats using a combination Hotz-Celsus and lateral eyelid wedge resection: results in 311 eyes. *Vet Ophthalmol*, **10** (1), 6–11.

See Appendix 2.

History

A 10-month-old male neutered Jack Russell Terrier is presented with a history of intermittent squinting and tearing for several weeks. The signs improved slightly with topical antibiotics but did not resolve. He has received routine vaccinations and anthelmintic treatment and is otherwise well.

Questions

1. Describe the abnormalities and pertinent normal features in Figs. 2.2a and b.
2. What differential diagnoses should be considered for this presentation?
3. What tests could you perform to make the diagnosis?

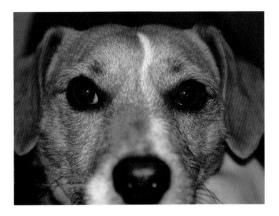

Fig. 2.2a

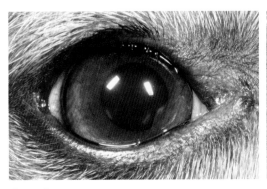 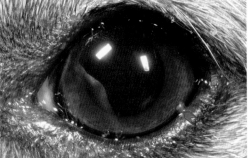

Fig. 2.2b

Answers

1. What the figures show

Fig. 2.2a There is a slightly narrowed palpebral fissure in the left eye compared with the right eye. **Fig. 2.2b** Both eyes are similar, the apparent anisocoria (OS < OD) represents a normal response to the ambient lighting conditions. There are several fine hairs along the upper and lower eyelid margins (OS > OD), some of which are coated with mucus (arrow). The leading edge of the third eyelid is non-pigmented. The Purkinje images are normal.

2. Differential diagnoses

Given the appearance of both eyes, the following conditions should be considered:

- **Distichiasis** This is a common condition in which extra eyelashes arise from the region of the meibomian glands and emerge from, or just posterior to, the gland openings along the eyelid margin (*Ch. 5, case 1, Diagram 5.1*). Distichiasis tends to occur in dogs less than one year old. It is often an incidental finding, but it can cause increased lacrimation, epiphora, and blepharospasm; corneal ulceration is uncommon. The degree of corneal irritation is related to the number, length and direction of the distichia. Short, stiff distichia tend to cause irritation whereas long, soft distichia cause little if any irritation unless they are present in high numbers and/or are directed towards the ocular surface. Distichia may act as a wick, causing tears to overflow onto the periocular hairs, mimicking a problem with tear drainage. Predisposed breeds are the Cocker Spaniel (American and English), Boxer, English Bulldog, Flat-Coated Retriever, Shih Tzu, Pekingese, Poodle, Dachsund and Jack Russell Terrier.
- **Ectopic cilia** This is a condition in which extra eyelashes arise from the region of the meibomian glands but, in contrast to distichiasis, emerge through the palpebral conjunctiva 4–6 mm from the eyelid margin. Ectopic cilia most commonly occur in the centre of the upper eyelid and cause direct irritation to the ocular surface (*Ch. 5, case 1, Diagram 5.1*). The typical clinical presentation is acute onset blepharospasm, lacrimation and corneal ulceration in a young dog (usually less than one year old). Clinical signs may be intermittent because ectopic cilia eventually fall out, only to regrow several weeks later. Predisposed breeds include the Lhasa Apso, Pekingese, Shih Tzu, Poodle, English Bulldog, Flat-Coated Retriever and Boxer (*Ch. 5, case 1*).
- **Trichiasis** This is a condition in which periocular hairs growing in a normal location are abnormally directed towards the ocular surface. If severe, trichiasis can cause conjunctivitis and keratitis, with associated discomfort. Trichiasis results from entropion and eyelid agenesis and can also be associated with nasal folds, medial canthus and caruncle.

3. Appropriate diagnostic tests

- Ocular reflexes
  - Pupillary light reflex – direct and consensual positive OU
  - Dazzle reflex – positive OU
  - Palpebral reflex – positive OU
- Menace response – positive OU
- Examination with a focal light source – slit-lamp biomicroscopy reveals that fine hairs emerge from the meibomian gland orifices along the eyelid margins, and that the upper and lower puncta are a normal size and shape in both eyes.
- Schirmer tear test – 27 mm/min OS, 22 mm/min OD. This is consistent with slightly increased lacrimation in the left eye.
- Fluorescein dye
  - Staining – negative OS, subtle positive staining ('stippling') OD. This is suggestive of minor disruption to the tear film in the right eye (Fig. 2.2c, A and B).

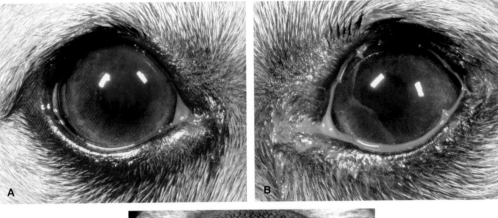

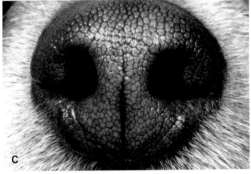

Fig. 2.2c (A) Fluorescein-positive 'stippling', right eye. (B) Wicking of fluorescein dye onto periocular hairs, left eye. (C) Negative Jones test on both sides.

- ○ Jones test (fluorescein dye passage test) – negative OU. This is consistent with reduced or absent tear drainage in both eyes (Fig. 2.2c, C).
- ○ Tear film break-up time – 20 s OU
- Tonometry – IOP 17 mmHg OU

The remainder of the ophthalmic examination reveals no additional abnormalities and a general physical examination is unremarkable.

Further diagnostic tests
Nasolacrimal cannulation and flush (performed under general anaesthesia) – flushing in a normograde direction (eye to nose) confirms the patency of the nasolacrimal system (Fig. 2.2d). The negative Jones test in both eyes demonstrates a reduced rate of tear drainage rather than obstruction of the nasolacrimal system.

Cannulation of the nasolacrimal punctum can be performed with a metal or plastic lacrimal cannula. The size of the cannula (22–25 gauge) depends on the size of the animal; plastic cannulas with an outer diameter of 0.9 mm in the dog and 0.76 mm in the cat are usually appropriate. Cutting the plastic cannula short and at an oblique angle facilitates cannulation. Intravenous catheters (with the metal stylet removed) can also be used. Sterile saline is usually used for flushing although tap water, distilled water and lactated Ringer's solution are acceptable alternatives. Cannulation of the upper punctum is generally preferred because it avoids the risk of inadvertent damage to the lower punctum which is responsible for the majority of tear drainage, and because it is usually easier.

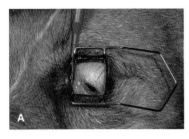
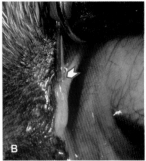
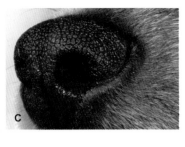

Fig. 2.2d Nasolacrimal flush under general anaesthesia. (A) and (B) Left upper nasolacrimal punctum (arrow) is cannulated with a plastic nasolacrimal cannula (outer diameter 0.76 mm). Saline is flushed initially to the lower punctum, which is then occluded by digital pressure, and then to the ipislateral nostril (C).

Diagnosis

Based on the information available, a diagnosis of distichiasis is made in both eyes. The epiphora in the left eye is a result of increased lacrimation overwhelming the nasolacrimal drainage system because of the greater number of distichia on that side.

Treatment

Most dogs with distichia do not require treatment. Treatment is only indicated if there are signs of ocular irritation. A topical lubricant, e.g. paraffin-based ointment, carbomer polymer gel, may be sufficient in cases of very mild irritation – the lubricant provides a layer in which the distichia 'float', minimising direct contact between the cilia and the cornea. Management of the condition by manual epilation with forceps following topical anaesthesia is generally unsuccessful, as the distichia re-grow. However, manual epilation can be useful to confirm that the cilia are the cause of the clinical signs. When treatment for distichiasis is indicated, surgical management is usually necessary. The aim of surgery is the permanent destruction or removal of the distichia hair follicles. Options include electroepilation, electrolysis, electrocautery, cryosurgery, radiohyperthermia and sharp dissection (partial resection of the distal tarsal plate, transpalpebral dissection and eyelid re-positioning techniques). There are limitations with all these techniques and, most importantly, all require general anaesthesia and magnification.

Cryosurgery is a popular technique performed by veterinary ophthamologists and is chosen for this dog. The eyelid is stabilised within a Desmarres chalazion clamp and everted to expose the palpebral conjunctiva near the eyelid margin. The cryotherapy handpiece is held in contact with the conjunctiva and a double freeze-thaw cycle is performed to freeze the tissue to −25°C (Fig. 2.2e). At this temperature the hair follicles should be destroyed but damage to the eyelid tissue is avoided. There are several appropriate cryogens, but nitrous oxide is generally used in veterinary medicine. Ideally, a thermocouple needle is inserted into the tissue to be treated but this is not routinely done in animals. Eyelid swelling can occur postoperatively and with some cryogens this can be so severe as to impair blinking (Fig. 2.2f). The swelling appears to cause little discomfort and usually subsides within two to three days. The eyelid margins and eyelid hairs can depigment within several days of treatment but generally repigment within a few months (Fig. 2.2g). Postoperative medication includes topical antibiotic-corticosteroid eye ointment and systemic NSAIDs.

Prognosis

The prognosis for improvement of the clinical signs following removal of distichia is good. The aim of treatment is to reduce the overall number of distichia to a level compatible with ocular comfort.

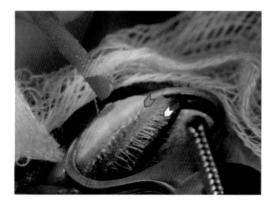

Fig. 2.2e Distichia (blue arrow); normal eyelashes (white arrow).

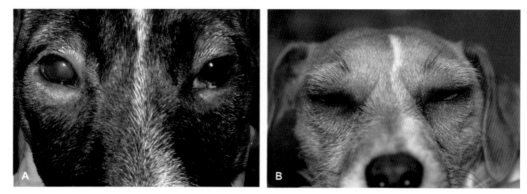

Fig. 2.2f (A) Immediate postoperative eyelid swelling in a young terrier with bilateral distichiasis treated with cryotherapy. (B) Severe immediate postoperative eyelid swelling in the dog from this case.

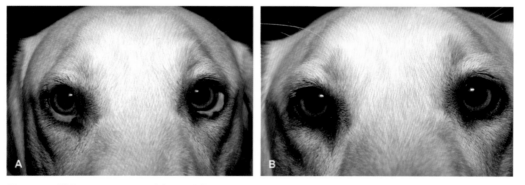

Fig. 2.2g (A) Depigmentation of the eyelid margin in a young Labrador one week after cryotherapy for bilateral distichiasis. (B) Repigmentation three months later.

Recurrence is possible with any of the techniques and repeated treatment is often necessary. Complications specific to cryotherapy include permanent depigmentation of the eyelid skin and hair (a cosmetic problem that is most relevant in show dogs). Excessive freezing of the eyelid can result in necrosis of the tissue and subsequent scarring and eyelid distortion, or damage to the meibomian glands which can result in a qualitative tear film abnormality.

Discussion

Distichiasis is a common condition in the dog and should only be treated if ocular discomfort is present because the techniques available are not entirely benign – the complications of treatment may be more significant than the initial condition. A thorough ophthalmic examination should be performed to ensure that the distichiasis is the primary cause of the clinical signs (*case 1, this chapter*). It is interesting to note that breeds predisposed to distichiasis also tend to be predisposed to ectopic cilia *(Ch. 5, case 1).*

Further reading

See Appendix 2.

History

A 3-year-old male neutered Shar Pei is presented with a six-month history of bilateral eyelid swellings and reduced vision. The dog has received routine vaccinations and regular anthelmintic treatment, and is otherwise clinically well.

Questions

1. Describe the abnormalities and pertinent normal features in Figs. 2.3a and b.
2. What differential diagnoses should be considered for this presentation?
3. What tests could you perform to make the diagnosis?

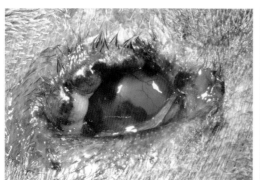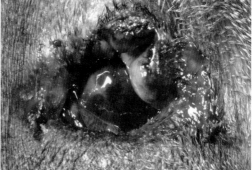

Fig. 2.3a

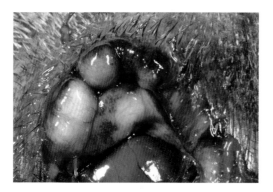

Fig. 2.3b

Answers

1. What the figures show

Fig. 2.3a The right and left eyes are similar. There is a moderate amount of mucoid discharge on the eyelid margins and eyelids. There is also hyperpigmentation and alopecia of the eyelid and periocular skin. The upper eyelids and their margins are distorted by multiple focal swellings; the lower eyelids are relatively normal. There is conjunctival hyperaemia and hyperpigmentation of the leading edge of the TEL and generalised corneal opacification and pigmentation. The ocular surface is lustrous but the distorted Purkinje images suggest that it is irregular. Corneal opacification prevents visualisation of the intraocular structures.

Fig. 2.3b Right eye – the upper eyelid has been manually everted for the purposes of demonstration. The focal swellings appear to be subconjunctival; these swellings are of different sizes and are tan coloured. The palpebral conjunctiva is pigmented in areas and is mildly hyperaemic; the pigmentation is indicative of chronic disease.

2. Differential diagnoses

Given the history and the appearance of both eyes, the following conditions should be considered for the eyelid abnormalities:

- **Inflammatory**
  - **Chalazion** This term describes a firm, non-painful swelling of the meibomian gland located adjacent to the eyelid margin. It is caused by obstruction of the duct of the gland which leads to accumulation of inspissated lipid secretions (meibum) and gland rupture. The liberated secretions causes a chronic granulomatous inflammatory reaction within the eyelid.
  - **Hordoleum or stye** An external hordoleum or stye develops from suppurative infection of the Zeiss or Moll glands located adjacent to the eyelid margin. A hordoleum appears as single or multiple abscesses along the eyelid margin. An internal hordoleum is caused by a localised infection within the tarsal plate and distends the palpebral conjunctiva. Both conditions are painful.
  - **Meibomianitis** This term refers to inflammation of the meibomian glands which causes lid swelling and discomfort. Chronic meibomianitis can result in thickened fibrotic eyelids and associated entropion or ectropion which may require surgical correction.
  - **Bacterial blepharitis** This can occur as part of juvenile pyoderma (or 'puppy strangles') in which multiple abscesses form on the head, including the eyelids. In the adult dog, *Staphylococcus* sp and *Streptococcus* sp can cause diffuse superficial blepharitis, pyogranulomatous blepharitis and meibomianitis.
  - **Blepharomycosis** This is uncommon and is usually part of a generalised skin problem in young dogs.
  - **Parasitic blepharitis** This is caused by demodectic and sarcoptic mange and is usually part of a generalised skin problem in young dogs. *Cuterebra* sp infestation (larva of the bot fly) is rare but can involve the conjunctiva and the eyelid.
  - **Protozoal blepharitis** Eyelid involvement is common with systemic leishmaniasis and signs include alopecia, diffuse blepharoedema, ulceration and discrete nodular granulomas.
  - **Immune-mediated blepharitis** Immune-mediated and auto-immune diseases can involve the eyelids, either in isolation or as part of a generalised disease process. Eyelid lesions are typically ulcerative in nature.
  - **Histiocytosis** This condition is seen primarily in the Bernese Mountain Dog and exists in two forms, a slow cutaneous form and a more aggressive malignant form with multi-organ involvement. Both forms can have eyelid involvement, e.g. chronic nodules, papules and plaques.

- ◦ **Nodular granulomatous episclerokeratitis (NGE)** NGE (or nodular ocular fasciitis) is an inflammatory condition manifested by the formation of a mass which primarily involves the episclera, conjunctiva and cornea (*Ch. 6, case 3*). Eyelids and third eyelids can be affected, and involvement of the uveal tract has also been described. The lesion can be single or multiple. Collies are predisposed.
- **Neoplasia** Eyelid neoplasia is common in the dog and benign neoplasms outnumber malignant neoplasms by 3:1. Most affected dogs are over 10 years old. Fibroma/fibrosarcoma, mastocytoma, lipoma, squamous cell carcinoma, histiocytoma, and papilloma of the eyelid have been described in the dog. The most common eyelid neoplasms are:
  - ◦ **Meibomian gland adenoma** The most common eyelid neoplasm in the dog which erupts through the eyelid margin or the palpebral conjunctiva. The mass can be pink or pigmented, lobular and can ulcerate, bleed and cause ocular surface irritation. A single mass is common but several masses may develop in the same individual. Meibomian gland adenocarcinomas are rare.
  - ◦ **Eyelid melanoma** The second most common eyelid neoplasm in the dog. Similar to other cutaneous melanomas, eyelid melanoma is usually benign but has a tendency to recur locally following excision.

3. Appropriate diagnostic tests

- Ocular reflexes
  - ◦ Pupillary light reflex – direct and consensual positive OU
  - ◦ Dazzle reflex – positive OU
  - ◦ Palpebral reflex – positive OU
  - ◦ Corneal reflex – positive OU
- Menace response – positive OU
- Examination with a focal light source – slit-lamp biomicroscopy reveals superficial corneal vascularisation and that the orifices of the meibomian glands are obscured by subconjunctival swellings.
- Ophthalmoscopy – fundic examination is limited by the corneal pathology but reveals no abnormalities in either eye.
- Schirmer tear test – 17 mm/min OU
- Fluorescein dye
  - ◦ Staining – negative OU
  - ◦ Jones test (fluorescein dye passage test) – positive OU
  - ◦ Tear film break-up time – approximately 5 s OU. This is consistent with reduced tear film stability in both eyes.
- Tonometry – IOP 20 mmHg OU

The remainder of the ophthalmic examination reveals no additional abnormalities and a general physical examination is unremarkable.

Diagnosis

A diagnosis of chalazia is made in both eyes. This is based on the lack of discomfort and the appearance of the lesions, specifically the tan colour and the association with the eyelid margins.

Treatment

Chalazia can be treated by curettage under general anaesthesia. To perform curettage, the eyelid is stabilised within a Desmarres chalazion clamp, and a scalpel blade incision is made into the con-

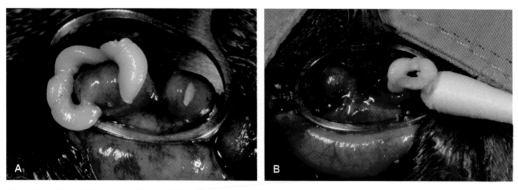

Fig. 2.3c (A) Stabilization of the right upper eyelid within a Desmarres chalazion clamp. Incisions have been made in the palpebral conjunctiva and the meibomian gland secretion has been partially expressed from the more lateral of the swellings. (B) Inspissated secretion from the meibomian gland (meibum) is expressed onto a sterile bacteriology swab.

junctiva overlying the swelling. The secretions can be gently expressed and samples taken and submitted for bacteriology (Fig. 2.3c). In this dog, each chalazion is gently curetted with a surgical curette and/or cannula to remove as much of the secretion as possible and the conjunctival incisions are left to heal by secondary intention.

In uncomplicated disease, a topical broad-spectrum antibiotic ointment is applied for approximately 10 days. In more severe cases, medical therapy following curettage often requires topical and systemic broad-spectrum antibiotic and systemic NSAID therapy for several weeks. A topical lacrimomimetic is indicated to address the qualitative tear film deficiency. Superficial keratitis is treated symptomatically with a topical anti-inflammatory agent, e.g. corticosteroid (dexamethasone), NSAID (ketorolac trometamol) or 0.2% cyclosporine. In addition to its lacrimostimulant effect (increasing the aqueous component of the tear film), cyclosporine increases mucin within the tear film and reduces corneal vascularisation and pigmentation. Treatment should be continued until the signs of keratitis show no further improvement, i.e. are stable – this may take weeks to months.

This dog receives a four-week course of carprofen, a six-week course of systemic oxytetracycline, a paraffin-based ophthalmic ointment, q8–12 hours for several weeks and 0.2% cyclosporine ointment q12 hours for three months, at which stage the corneal vascularisation and pigmentation are considered to be stable.

Prognosis

The prognosis for the resolution of chalazia is good with appropriate surgical and medical management. There is complete resolution of the chalazia six weeks following treatment in this dog (Fig. 2.3d).

Discussion

A chalazion is a common eyelid condition in the dog but this case is unusual because of the size and number of chalazia, the bilateral symmetry and the secondary superficial keratitis. The meibomian glands secrete meibum, an essential lipid component of the tear film, which reduces tear evaporation. Disease of the meibomian glands can therefore result in a qualitative tear film

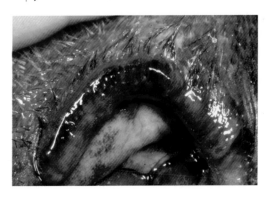

Fig. 2.3d Right upper eyelid six weeks following surgical curettage and medical management. The chalazia have resolved and the eyelid margin appears more normal, albeit slightly thickened. The conjunctival and corneal changes remain unchanged.

abnormality. The diagnosis of qualitative tear film disorders in the dog can be challenging, not least because they are infrequent compared to a quantitative tear film deficiency (keratoconjunctivitis sicca). A qualitative tear film disorder can involve the lipid or the mucin layers of the tear film and should be suspected if there is ocular surface disease in the presence of normal aqueous tear production (i.e. a normal STT value). Measurement of the tear film break-up time is often beneficial.

Tear film break-up time (TBUT) is a measure of the stability of the tear film. TBUT is a measure of the time taken for the tear film to dissociate from the ocular surface. Fluorescein dye is applied to the ocular surface, the eye is allowed to blink and then the eyelids are held open. The time is takes for the first dark spot to appear in the tear film is measured. This procedure is facilitated by slit-lamp biomicroscopy and a cobalt-blue filter. The average TBUT is 20 s in the dog and 16.7 s in the cat.

Further reading
See Appendix 2.

CHAPTER 3

Abnormalities of the Third Eyelid

Introduction

The third eyelid (TEL) has an important role in the health of the ocular surface because the gland of the TEL contributes to the aqueous portion of the precorneal tear film. The TEL can also be involved in the distribution of the tear film. The position of the TEL is closely related to the size and position of the eye and a change in position and appearance of the TEL provides information about abnormalities of the globe and the orbit. Regardless of the underlying condition, protrusion of the TEL is a common reason for presentation.

Small Animal Ophthalmology: What's Your Diagnosis? First Edition. Heidi Featherstone, Elaine Holt.
© 2011 by Heidi Featherstone and Elaine Holt. Published 2011 by Blackwell Publishing Ltd.

History

A 1-year-old female neutered Beagle is presented because of a swelling in the corner of each eye. The swelling in the left eye has been present for several weeks but has not appeared to cause discomfort; the swelling in the right eye has only been present for three weeks. The dog has received routine vaccinations and anthelmintic treatment and is reportedly to be clinically well.

Questions

1. Describe the abnormalities and pertinent normal features in Figs. 3.1a and b.
2. What differential diagnoses should be considered for this presentation?
3. What tests could you perform to make the diagnosis?

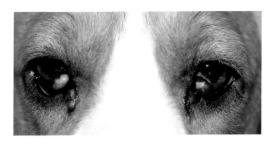

Fig. 3.1a

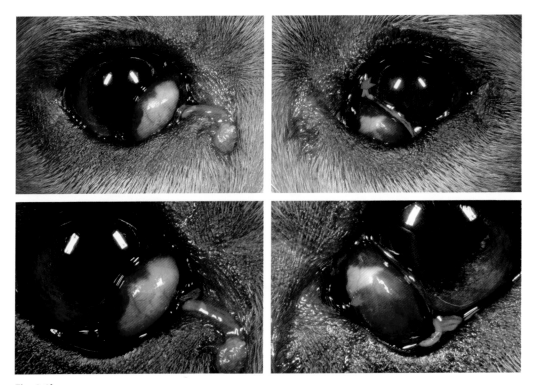

Fig. 3.1b

Answers

1. What the figures show
Figs. 3.1a and b Both eyes are similar. A smooth, oval pink-to-brown mass protrudes from behind the TEL (arrows). There is a seromucoid discharge at the medial canthus in the right eye and along the edge of the mass in the left eye.

2. Differential diagnoses
Given the appearance of both eyes, the following conditions should be considered:

- **Prolapse of the gland of the TEL ('cherry eye')** This is the most common primary disorder of the TEL in the dog. The condition is thought to result from a weakness in the connective tissue attachment between the gland of the TEL and the periorbital tissue. The gland detaches and becomes visible above the leading edge of the TEL as a smooth pink mass. The condition can be unilateral or bilateral and usually occurs before two years of age. It is common in the Cocker Spaniel (American and English), Beagle and brachycephalic dog breeds such as the Lhasa Apso, English Bulldog and Pekingese, as well as large and giant dog breeds such as the Great Dane and Mastiff.

- **Scrolled cartilage of the TEL** Eversion, or less commonly inversion, of the T-shaped cartilage within the TEL leads to folding of the leading edge of the TEL and exposure of the bulbar surface (Fig. 3.1c). The proximal portion of the upright stem of the cartilage is usually affected. Most commonly seen in young, large-dog breeds, it is thought to occur because of a differential rate of growth between the posterior and anterior portions of the cartilage. The condition can be associated with poor distribution of the tear film, chronic low-grade ocular surface irritation, and conjunctivitis.

- **Neoplasia** Neoplasia of the TEL is uncommon in the dog. Several neoplasms have been reported and include adenocarcinoma of the TEL gland, papilloma and malignant melanoma. Adenocarcinoma of the TEL gland can appear as a localised, firm, pink swelling on the bulbar surface of the TEL and as such must be differentiated from prolapse of the TEL gland; more advanced tumours can present as orbital disease. Adenocarcinomas usually occur in middle-aged to older dogs. TEL papillomas are benign cauliflower-like growths from the conjunctival surface whereas TEL melanomas are usually malignant and appear as brown to black lesions on the conjunctiva.

- **Conjunctival cyst** This is an uncommon condition in the dog with multiple forms. Congenital/developmental epithelial inclusion cysts, parasitic cysts, cystic neoplasia, and cysts of the gland of the TEL, lacrimal gland (dacryops), and canaliculi (canaliculops) have been described. Cysts are usually slow-growing, non-painful conjunctival swellings.

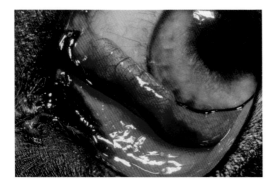

Fig. 3.1c Eversion of the leading edge of the TEL in the left eye of a young Great Dane.

- **Subconjunctival fat prolapse** Prolapse of orbital fat appears as a non-painful, slightly moveable subconjunctival mass adjacent to the limbus.

3. Appropriate diagnostic tests
- Ocular reflexes
  - Pupillary light reflex – direct and consensual positive OU
  - Dazzle reflex – positive OU
- Menace response – positive OU
- Schirmer tear test – 22 mm/min OU
- Fluorescein dye
  - Staining – negative OU
  - Jones test (fluorescein dye passage test) – positive OU
- Tonometry – IOP 15 mmHg OU

Following topical anaesthesia, manipulation of the TEL with atraumatic forceps in both eyes confirms that the swellings are associated with the bulbar surface of the TEL and do not involve the leading edge. The remainder of the ophthalmic examination reveals no additional abnormalities and a general physical examination is unremarkable.

> Atraumatic forceps can be used to manipulate the TEL in the conscious animal. Graefe fixation forceps and Bennett cilia forceps are particularly useful and avoid inadvertent damage to the TEL.

Diagnosis
Based on the information available, a diagnosis of bilateral prolapse of the gland of the TEL is made. In this dog the conjunctiva covering the gland is pigmented – this is an unusual finding and is considered to be the result of chronic exposure.

Treatment
Until the mid-1970s, surgical excision of the prolapsed gland was considered an acceptable treatment but the important role of the gland of the TEL in tear production has since been recognised and surgery to reposition the gland is currently strongly advised. Without treatment the prolapsed gland can become enlarged and inflamed, resulting in chronic conjunctivitis, irritation and ocular discharge. There are several published techniques to surgically reposition the gland and these techniques can be divided into those that anchor the gland in position and those that create a conjunctival pocket for the gland. There is currently no published information that compares the different techniques with regard to their effect on tear production or the potential for the gland to re-prolapse following surgery.

The Morgan pocket technique is chosen and used in this dog. After induction of general anaesthesia but prior to the start of the surgery, one drop of topical 2.5% phenylephrine is applied to the ocular surface (Fig. 3.1d). Two parallel curvilinear incisions are made in the bulbar conjunctiva, one either side of the gland (Fig. 3.1e). Following blunt dissection to create a pocket beneath the most distal incision, the gland is reduced into this area of dead space. The conjunctival wound is closed with a simple continuous pattern of 6/0 absorbable suture material (polyglactin 910), leaving both knots on the anterior surface of the TEL. Postoperative medication includes a five-day course of systemic NSAID and broad-spectrum antibiotic therapy, and a topical steroid/antibiotic preparation which is administered for 14 days.

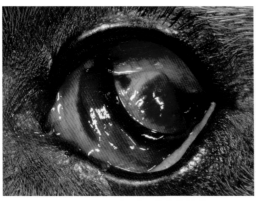

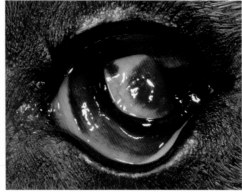

Fig. 3.1d Blanching of the conjunctival vasculature because of vasoconstriction following the topical application of 2.5% phenylephrine in the left eye.

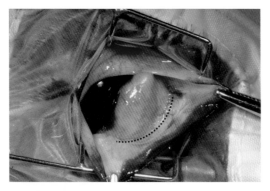

Fig. 3.1e Intraoperative photograph of the posterior aspect of the TEL, revealing the prolapsed gland and the position of the conjunctival incision above the gland (dotted line).

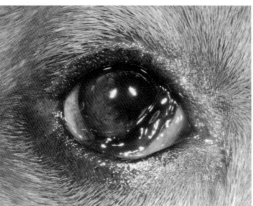

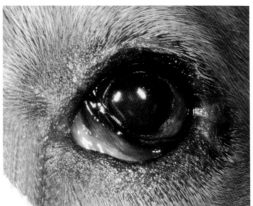

Fig. 3.1f Postoperative appearance at two hours. The TELs are slightly more prominent than usual and there is mild chemosis and conjunctival hyperaemia – expected findings at this stage.

The topical application of 2.5% phenylephrine causes local vasoconstriction and can minimise intraoperative haemorrhage during surgery which involves the conjunctiva and the TEL. The phenylephrine should be applied <u>before</u> an incision is made. This should help to avoid direct arterial and venous access, which could lead to unwanted systemic effects on the heart rate and blood pressure (Herring *et al.*, 2004).

Prognosis

Proper surgical technique, adequate magnification and illumination, and appropriate instrumentation should result in successful replacement of the gland and a good cosmetic outcome (Fig. 3.1f). One study reports that the rate of re-prolapse following the Morgan pocket technique is significantly lower than with anchoring techniques whilst other studies report a low rate of

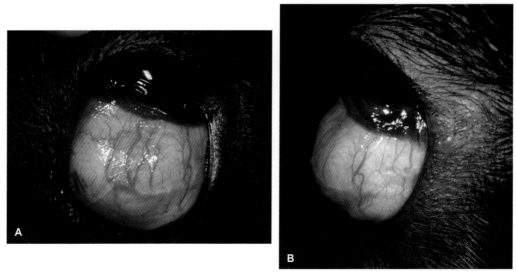

Fig. 3.1g Large cyst within the TEL of a young Rottweiler one month following the Morgan pocket technique to replace a prolapsed gland of the TEL (left eye). (A) Frontal view. (B) Oblique view.

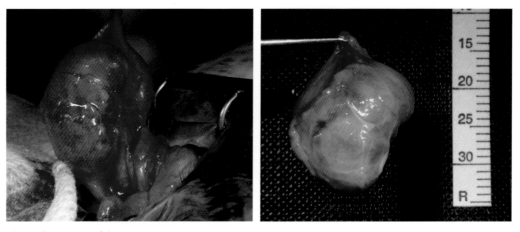

Fig. 3.1h Excision of the intact cyst.

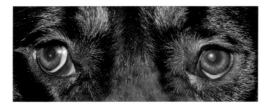

Fig. 3.1i Ten days following excision of the cyst from the left TEL.

re-prolapse (0–4%) following anchoring techniques (Moore and Constantinescu, 1997). Postoperative complications include cyst formation, suture reaction, corneal ulceration (as a result of exposed suture material contacting the ocular surface) and reduced mobility of the TEL. Cyst formation following the pocket technique is thought to occur if the conjunctival incision is closed without leaving a small gap at either end for the escape of tear secretions. A cyst will typically form several weeks after surgery and presents as a non-painful swelling of the TEL; this is often misinterpreted by the owner as re-prolapse of the gland (Fig. 3.1g). Cysts can be surgically excised intact (Fig. 3.1h) resulting in a good cosmetic outcome (Fig. 3.1i).

Discussion

Although re-positioning of the TEL gland preserves its tear function, it is still possible for an affected eye to develop keratoconjunctivitis sicca (KCS) for other reasons. The reason for this is that many breeds predisposed to prolapse of the TEL gland are also predisposed to immune-mediated KCS.

It is generally accepted by veterinary ophthalmologists that the Mastiff and Mastiff-type breeds have a greater likelihood of complications following TEL gland surgery than other dog breeds. These breeds often have marked hypertrophy of the gland and inflammation of the overlying conjunctiva at presentation, both of which can lead to more challenging surgery.

References and further reading

Herring IP, Jacobson JD, Pickett JP (2004) Cardiovascular effects of topical ophthalmic 10% phenylephrine in dogs. *Vet Ophthalmol*, **7**(1), 41–46.

Moore CP & Constantinescu GM (1997) Surgery of the adnexa. *Vet Clin North Am Small Animal Pract*, **27**(5), 1052–1058.

See Appendix 2.

History

A 3-year-old male German Shepherd Dog is presented because of red eyes and a sticky ocular discharge for several weeks. The dog has received routine vaccinations and anthelmintic treatment and is reported to be clinically well.

Questions

1. Describe the abnormalities and pertinent normal features in Figs. 3.2a and 3.2b.
2. What differential diagnoses should be considered for this presentation?
3. What tests could you perform to make the diagnosis?

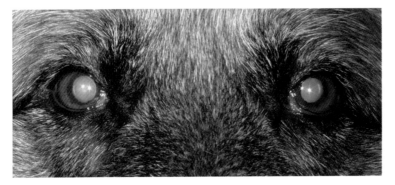

Fig. 3.2a

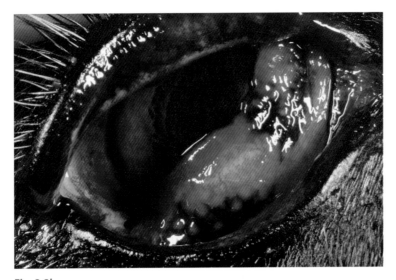

Fig. 3.2b

Answers

1. What the figures show

Fig. 3.2a The left and right eyes are similar. There is a mild increased prominence of the TEL (OS > OD) and hyperaemia of the TEL conjunctiva. The tapetal reflection is opalescent because of nuclear sclerosis. The Purkinje images are normal. Right eye – fluorescein dye is visible within the tear film meniscus along the lower eyelid.

Fig. 3.2b Only the right eye is shown. The upper eyelid has been manually everted and the globe retropulsed so that the TEL can be evaluated. The leading edge of the TEL is irregular and there are multiple lymphoid follicles on the anterior aspect of TEL which appear as small, round, pink nodules. There is hyperaemia and depigmentation of the TEL, bulbar and palpebral conjunctivae. The lustrous cornea suggests the presence of an adequate tear film.

2. Differential diagnoses

Given the appearance of both TELs, the following conditions should be considered:

- **Plasma cell infiltration of the TEL (atypical pannus or 'plasmoma')** This appears as thickening and depigmentation of the TEL associated with follicle formation. Plasma cell infiltration of the TEL is often associated with chronic superficial keratitis (pannus) but can also occur in isolation. The condition is usually bilateral and the German Shepherd Dog is predisposed. A conjunctival inflammatory infiltrate consisting predominantly of plasma cells and fewer lymphocytes is seen on histopathology.
- **Follicular conjunctivitis** Lymphoid follicles on the bulbar surface of the TEL are normal but in follicular conjunctivitis the follicles are larger and more numerous and can also form on the palpebral surface. Follicular conjunctivitis can cause mild protrusion of the TEL and a mucoid discharge. Large dog breeds and dogs less than 18 months old are most commonly affected. The cause is unknown but it is thought to be because of chronic antigenic stimulation.
- **Nodular granulomatous episclerokeratitis (NGE)** NGE (or ocular nodular fasciitis) is an inflammatory condition which primarily involves the episclera, conjunctiva and cornea. The clinical appearance ranges from an irregular thickening to a discrete mass or nodule, most commonly at the dorsolateral region of the limbus. The eyelids and TEL can be involved; if affected the TEL is hyperaemic, thickened and depigmented. Involvement of the uveal tract has also been described. A mixed inflammatory infiltrate composed predominantly of lymphocytes, plasma cells and histiocytes with a variable spindle cell component is seen on histopathology. Collies are predisposed.
- **Idiopathic granulomatous disease** This is an inflammatory condition which is characterised by multiple masses involving the eyelids, conjunctiva, TEL and skin. Granulomatous inflammation with large epithelioid cells, plasma cells and lymphocytes is seen on histopathology.
- **Neoplasia** Neoplasia of the TEL is uncommon in the dog. Several neoplasms have been reported and include adenocarcinoma of the TEL gland, papilloma and malignant melanoma. Adenocarcinoma of the TEL gland can appear as a localised, firm, pink swelling on the bulbar surface of the TEL and as such must be differentiated from TEL gland prolapse; more advanced tumours can present as orbital disease. Adenocarcinomas usually occur in middle-aged to older dogs. TEL papillomas are benign cauliflower-like growths from the conjunctival surface whereas TEL melanomas are usually malignant and appear as brown to black lesions on the conjunctiva. Less common TEL neoplasms include squamous cell carcinoma and lymphosarcoma; the latter may be bilateral and manifests as thickening and hyperaemia of the TEL.

3. Appropriate diagnostic tests

- Ocular reflexes
  - ○ Pupillary light reflex – direct and consensual positive OU
  - ○ Dazzle reflex – positive OU
- Menace response – positive OU
- Schirmer tear test – 20 mm/min OU
- Fluorescein dye – negative staining OU
- Cytology and biopsy – these tests are not performed in this dog because of the characteristic appearance but can be helpful to distinguish an inflammatory from a neoplastic process.

The remainder of the ophthalmic examination reveals no additional abnormalities and a general physical examination is unremarkable.

Diagnosis

Based on the information available, a diagnosis of bilateral plasma cell infiltration of the TEL is made. This diagnosis is usually based on the classic appearance of the TEL in the age and breed of dog without the need for conjunctival cytology or histopathology.

Treatment

Treatment of plasma cell infiltration of the TEL is usually based on topical immunosuppressive therapy. Corticosteroids are the mainstay of therapy and 0.1% prednisolone acetate or 0.1% dexamethasone sodium phosphate are the drugs of choice. The frequency of application depends on the severity of the clinical signs and may range from q4–12 hours. The frequency should be tapered over weeks as the inflammation decreases. Cyclosporine A (0.2% ointment, or drops up to 2%) can also be used q12 hours; it tends to be more expensive and may not be as effective as corticosteroid therapy in achieving remission, but can be beneficial for long-term maintenance therapy. A sub-conjunctival injection of a long-acting corticosteroid (e.g. triamcinolone) can be considered in refractory cases or in dogs that do not tolerate topical treatment.

This dog receives 0.1% dexamethasone sodium phosphate q6 hours for 10 days and then q8 hours until re-examination three months later (Fig. 3.2c). Frequency of drug application is decreased after 10 days because the conjunctival hyperaemia has improved, follicles are less prominent and there is subtle repigmentation. After three months, the leading edge of the TEL is more regular, the conjunctival hypaeremia has resolved and there is further repigmentation. The frequency of treatment is reduced to q12 hours and the dog monitored for signs of recurrence on a regular long-term basis.

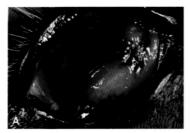 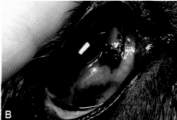 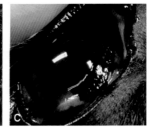

Fig. 3.2c (A) TEL at presentation. (B) Ten days after the start of topical treatment. (C) Three months after the start of topical treatment. There is a progressive reduction in conjunctival hypaeremia and number of follicles, conjunctival repigmentation and a smoothing of the leading edge of the TEL.

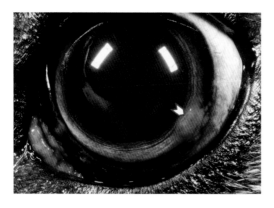

Fig. 3.2d Mild chronic superficial keratitis (arrow) in the ventrolateral quadrant of the left eye of a young German Shepherd Dog, in conjunction with plasma cell infiltration of the TEL.

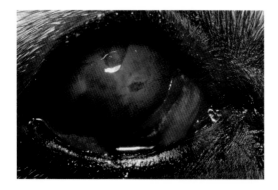

Fig. 3.2e Advanced chronic superficial keratitis in the right eye of a German Shepherd Dog – the entire cornea is vascularised, pigmented and fibrotic. There is plasma cell infiltration of the TEL.

Prognosis

The prognosis for the resolution of clinical signs is good, as most dogs with plasma cell infiltration of the TEL respond to appropriate topical therapy. It is, however, not uncommon for the resolution to be partial. Recurrence is common and long-term monitoring is important as most affected dogs require maintenance therapy for life, e.g. topical corticosteroid therapy or cyclosporine A q12–24 hours.

Discussion

Although plasma cell infiltration of the TEL can occur in isolation, it occurs more often in conjunction with chronic superficial keratitis (pannus). Chronic superficial keratitis begins as a vascular lesion in the conjunctiva near the lateral limbus, and can extend onto the adjacent cornea (Fig. 3.2d). Similar changes can occur at the medial aspect of the limbus and the entire cornea may eventually become vascularised and pigmented (Fig. 3.2e).

The syndrome of chronic superficial keratitis and plasma cell infiltration of the TEL is thought to be the result of an immune-mediated process. Chronic superficial keratitis is exacerbated by environmental factors such as ultraviolet radiation and altitude. The cornea contains tissue-specific antigens that are modified by external factors such as ultraviolet light resulting in cell-mediated inflammation. As with plasma cell infiltration of the TEL, the diagnosis of chronic superficial keratitis is usually based on the signalment and the clinical appearance.

Further reading

See Appendix 2.

History

A one-year-old female neutered Labrador Retriever is presented with a one-month history of lethargy and coughing, and asymmetry between the eyes over the last two weeks. The dog has received routine vaccinations and anthelmintic treatment.

Questions

1. Describe the abnormalities and pertinent normal features in Fig. 3.3a (A) on presentation and Figs. 3.3a (B) and 3.3b, 10 days later.
2. What differential diagnoses should be considered for this presentation?
3. What tests could you perform to make the diagnosis?

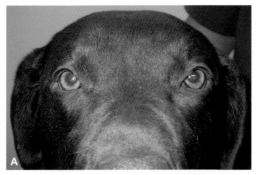

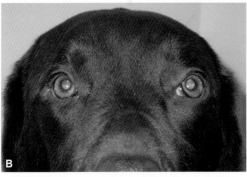

Fig. 3.3a (A) Initial presentation. (B) Ten days later.

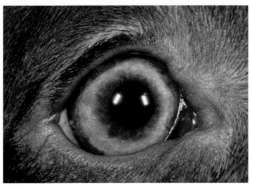

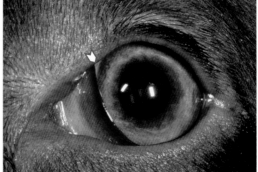

Fig. 3.3b

Answers

1. What the figures show
Fig. 3.3a Photograph B was taken 10 days after photograph A. The tapetal reflections are yellow in B but not discernable in A – this is because of a subtle difference in the direction of gaze. The right eye is normal. Left eye – there is subtle protrusion of the TEL which is more pronounced in B.

Fig. 3.3b Left eye – there is mild exotropia (lateral strabismus) evident by an increase in the amount of visible sclera on the medial aspect of the globe and reduced scleral show laterally. There is relative anisocoria (OS > OD) because of different ambient room light.

> Examination from a distance (as indicated in Fig. 3.3a) is essential in order to observe subtle asymmetry. If possible, restraint should be minimal so that the periocular skin is not disturbed and distortion of the palpebral fissure does not occur.

2. Differential diagnoses
Given the history and the appearance of the left eye, the following explanations should be considered:

- **Increased volume of orbital tissue** This can cause exophthalmos and/or strabismus and TEL protrusion. Causes include orbital inflammation, infection, neoplasia, cysts, immune-mediated disease and haemorrhage (*Ch. 1, case 3*).
- **Reduced orbital tissue volume** This results in enophthalmos and TEL protrusion. Causes include dehydration, marked weight loss (reduction of orbital fat) and fibrosis of orbital tissues following orbital inflammation or surgery.
- **Pain** Ocular surface pain and intraocular pain can lead to retraction of the globe and subsequent enophthalmos and protrusion of the TEL. Causes of ocular surface pain include disorders of the adnexa, tear film, conjunctiva, and cornea (*Ch. 2 and 5*). Causes of intraocular pain include uveitis and glaucoma (*Ch. 2, 6 and 7*).
- **Decreased tone of extraocular muscles** Horner's syndrome (*Ch. 10, case 1*) and some sedatives, e.g. acepromazine, cause enophthalmos as a result of decreased tone in the extraocular muscles.
- **Increased tone of extraocular muscles** Tetanus and strychnine poisoning cause TEL protrusion by increasing tone in the extraocular muscles.

> The TEL in the dog is devoid of muscle and its movement and position is determined by the position and size of the eye. In contrast, the TEL in the cat contains several muscles and its movement can be both active and passive.

3. Appropriate diagnostic tests
- Ocular reflexes
  - Pupillary light reflex – direct and consensual positive OU
  - Dazzle reflex – positive OU
  - Vestibulo-ocular reflex – positive OU
- Menace response – positive OU
- Schirmer tear test – 20 mm/min OU
- Fluorescein dye – negative staining OU
- Tonometry – IOP 18 mmHg OU

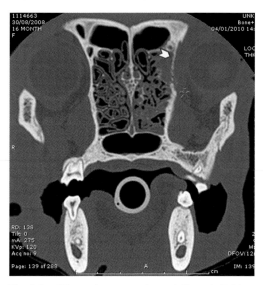

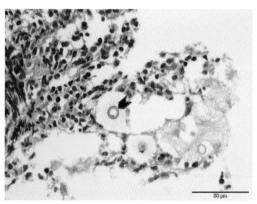

Fig. 3.3d Yeast organism (arrow) surrounded by clear space (capsule/shrinkage artefact). H & E stain (×400). Bar = 50 μm. Reproduced with permission from EJ Scurrell.

Fig. 3.3c CT scan (transverse image). There is fluid accumulation in the left nasal cavity, patchy lysis of the frontal bone of the medial orbit (arrow), and a soft tissue mass within the medial orbit (asterix).

Retropulsion is reduced and associated with pain in the left eye but is normal in the right eye. Examination of the bulbar aspect of the TEL in the left eye is performed following topical anaesthesia and reveals no abnormalities. The remainder of the ophthalmic examination and a general physical examination is unremarkable.

Further diagnostic tests
- Laboratory tests – routine haematology, biochemistry and urine analysis are unremarkable.
- CT scan – this is indicated to evaluate the orbit and adjacent structures. The scan reveals fluid accumulation in the left nasal cavity, patchy lysis of the frontal bone of the medial orbit (arrow), and a soft tissue mass within the medial orbit (asterix) (Fig. 3.3c).
- Cytology – FNA of the orbital mass is performed under ultrasound guidance; results are non-diagnostic.
- Rhinoscopy – this confirms the presence of fluid within the left nasal cavity and reveals several white plaques on the soft palate, from which multiple tissue biopsies are taken.
- Histopathology – small numbers of yeast organisms, surrounded by a thick capsule, can be seen, with an associated mixed inflammatory infiltrate. The appearance of the yeast organisms is typical for *Cryptococcus* sp (Fig. 3.3d).
- Serology – a latex agglutination antigen test for *Crypotoccosis neoformans* reveals a high titre of 1:2054.

Diagnosis
Based on the information available, a diagnosis of orbital cryptococcosis with systemic involvement is made.

Treatment
Anti-fungal therapy with fluconazole is considered the first line of treatment in dogs with ocular and central nervous system (CNS) cryptococcosis. The dose is 5 mg/kg *per os* q12–24 hours for

60–90 days. Amphotericin B has also been used alone and in combination with systemic anti-fungal therapy. The dose for amphotericin B is 0.5–0.8 mg/kg (diluted in 0.45% saline containing 2.5% dextrose) and is administered by subcutaneous injection two to three times weekly. Response to treatment should be monitored at least monthly by evaluation of antigen titres and renal and hepatic function. Treatment is continued until the antigen titre is negative and for at least two months after resolution of clinical signs.

This dog receives combination therapy of fluconazole and amphotericin B; there is excellent clinical improvement and the antigen titre decreases to 1:504 during the first month of treatment.

Prognosis

The prognosis for cryptococcosis is guarded because of the likelihood of CNS involvement. Serial evaluation of the antigen titre is not helpful for determining the prognosis but an initial decline in the titre by 25–50% per month usually corresponds to clinical improvement.

Discussion

Two subspecies have been recognised in dogs with cryptococcosis. *Cryptococcus neoformans* var. *neoformans* is associated with bird droppings and *C neoformans* var. *gattii*, is associated with eucalyptus trees. In tissues, the appearance is of a yeast-like organism with a thick capsule, with the size varying from 3.5–7 μm. Young (less than four years), medium to large dogs are most typically infected. Infection usually occurs via inhalation of spores with subsequent systemic dissemination. Clinical signs depend on the organ system(s) involved. In the dog, CNS (50–80%), upper respiratory system (50%), eye/orbit (20–40%) and skin (10–20%) involvement are most common. Non-specific clinical signs include anorexia, lethargy and depression. The most common ocular signs are chorioretinitis with exudative retinal detachment and optic neuritis because of leptomeningitis of the optic nerve. Diagnosis is made on the basis of cytology, histology, culture and serology. Canine cryptococcosis is less frequently diagnosed than feline cryptococcosis and is most often found in dogs from the southern US, Australia (in association with eucalyptus trees) and Canada (in association with fir trees).

References and further reading

Krohne SG (2000) Canine systemic fungal infections. *Vet Clin North Am: Small Animal Pract*, **30** (5) 1063–1090.

Duncan TBC (2006) Evaluation of risk factors for *Cryptococcus gattii* infection in dogs and cats. *J Am Vet Med Assoc*, **228** (3) 377–382.

See Appendix 2.

CHAPTER 4

Ocular Discharge

Introduction

Ocular discharge is a common presenting clinical sign in the dog and cat. The nature of the discharge can provide helpful information about the underlying problem, although the colour, consistency and amount of discharge are not specific to particular ocular conditions.

Small Animal Ophthalmology: What's Your Diagnosis? First Edition. Heidi Featherstone, Elaine Holt.
© 2011 by Heidi Featherstone and Elaine Holt. Published 2011 by Blackwell Publishing Ltd.

History

A 10-month-old female neutered Labrador Retriever is presented because of a watery discharge and the appearance of a swelling in the corner of the right eye. There are no apparent signs of discomfort. She has received routine vaccinations and anthelmintic treatment and is otherwise well.

Questions

1. Describe the abnormalities and pertinent normal features in Fig. 4.1a.
2. What differential diagnoses should be considered for this presentation?
3. What tests could you perform to make the diagnosis?

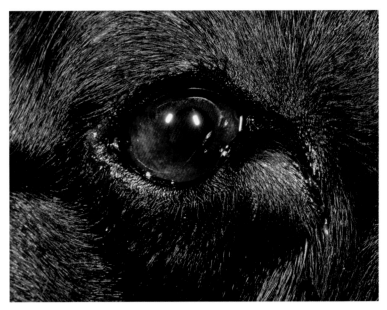

Fig. 4.1a

Answers

1. What does the figure show?

Fig. 4.1a Right eye – there is epiphora and a well-circumscribed swelling ventral to the medial canthus. A thin strand of mucus is adherent to the cornea; the Purkinje images are normal.

2. Differential diagnoses

Given the presence of epiphora and concurrent medial canthal swelling, the following conditions/ explanations should be considered:

- **Impaired tear drainage**
  - **Cyst** Congenital cysts can involve the canaliculus (canaliculops), and the nasolacrimal sac or duct (dacryops) as well as adjacent structures. A unilateral, non-painful swelling with epiphora in a young dog is a common presentation for this condition.
  - **Lacrimal punctal atresia** This is the most common congenital anomaly of the nasolacrimal system. It can be unilateral or bilateral and can affect the upper and/or lower punctum. Atresia of the upper punctum is usually asymptomatic because the majority of tear drainage occurs via the lower punctum. Clinical signs include epiphora, conjunctivitis and, if severe, secondary dermatitis involving the medial canthus and adjacent facial skin.
  - **Micropunctum** This refers to the incomplete development of the upper and/or lower punctum which appears as a small round opening rather than the normal elliptical opening (1×0.3 mm). It can be unilateral or bilateral and, as with upper punctal atresia, incomplete development of the upper punctum is usually asymptomatic. Clinical signs include epiphora and less frequently conjunctivitis.
  - **Misplaced punctum and canaliculus** This is an uncommon anomaly which is usually asymptomatic but can cause epiphora.
  - **Canalicular and nasolacrimal duct aplasia** Aplasia of the components of the nasolacrimal system other than the puncta are rare but if present can cause epiphora.
  - **Breed-related medial canthal anomalies** Compression of the lower punctum and canaliculus can result from lower medial entropion. Caruncular trichiasis and deep medial canthal grooves caused by tight medial canthal ligaments exacerbate the effects of the entropion. This syndrome is common in brachycephalic and small and toy breeds such as the Miniature and Toy Poodle and the Bichon Frisé. The clinical presentation varies in severity from mild bilateral epiphora to marked tear staining with secondary dermatitis (Fig. 4.1b).
  - **Dacryocystitis** Inflammation of the nasolacrimal sac is common condition in the dog and is usually caused by the presence of a foreign body lodged in the nasolacrimal sac or duct. Clinical

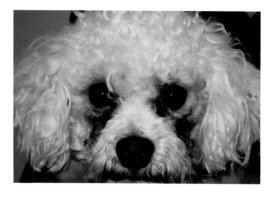

Fig. 4.1b Marked epiphora in a young Bichon Frisé secondary to compression of the lower puncta by medial lower entropion, and exacerbated by caruncular trichiasis and deep medial canthal grooves.

signs include epiphora, purulent ocular discharge, conjunctivitis, discomfort and, occasionally, a draining fistula ventral to the medial canthus.

- ○ **Facial trauma** Sharp trauma and fractures of the maxillary and lacrimal bones can damage the nasolacrimal duct system and cause epiphora.
- ○ **Neoplasia** Primary neoplasia of the nasolacrimal duct has not been reported in any species but nasal tumours can extend locally and compress or invade the nasolacrimal duct. Clinical signs include sneezing, mucopurulent or haemorrhagic nasal discharge and epiphora.
- **Increased lacrimation** This can result from either ocular surface or intraocular pain. The ocular surface is primarily innervated by the ophthalmic branch of the trigeminal nerve, with some contribution from the maxillary branch. Increased lacrimation overwhelms the nasolacrimal drainage system and epiphora results.

3. Appropriate diagnostic tests

- Ocular reflexes
  - ○ Pupillary light reflex – direct and consensual positive OU
  - ○ Dazzle reflex – positive OU
  - ○ Palpebral reflex – positive OU
- Menace response – positive OU
- Examination with a focal light source – slit-lamp biomicroscopy reveals that both upper and lower puncta are a normal size and shape OU.
- Schirmer tear test – 17 mm/min OS, 19 mm/min OD. These normal values suggest that there is reduced tear drainage rather than increased lacrimation in the right eye.
- Fluorescein dye
  - ○ Staining – negative OU
  - ○ Jones test (fluorescein dye passage test) – positive OS, negative OD. This finding supports reduced tear drainage on the right side (Fig. 4.1c).
- Tonometry – IOP 17 mmHg OU

The remainder of the ophthalmic examination reveals no additional abnormalities and a general physical examination is unremarkable.

Further diagnostic tests

- Nasolacrimal duct cannulation and flush (performed under general anaesthesia) – a normograde flush (eye to nose) confirms the patency of the nasolacrimal system in both eyes.

Cannulation of the nasolacrimal punctum can be performed with a metal or plastic lacrimal cannula. The size of the cannula (22–25 gauge) depends on the size of the animal; plastic cannulas with an outer diameter of 0.9 mm in the dog and 0.76 mm in the cat are usually appropriate. Cutting the plastic cannula short and at an oblique angle facilitates cannulation. Intravenous catheters (with the metal stylet removed) can also be used. Sterile saline is usually used for flushing although tap water, distilled water and lactated Ringer's solution are acceptable alternatives. Cannulation of the upper punctum is generally preferred because it avoids the risk of inadvertent damage to the lower punctum which is responsible for the majority of tear drainage, and because it is usually easier.

- Radiography – radiographic evaluation of the nasolacrimal system requires plain radiography followed by a contrast study (dacryocystorhinography). Following cannulation, radiopaque contrast material is injected into the upper punctum until it emerges from the ipsilateral nostril (1–2 ml in the dog).

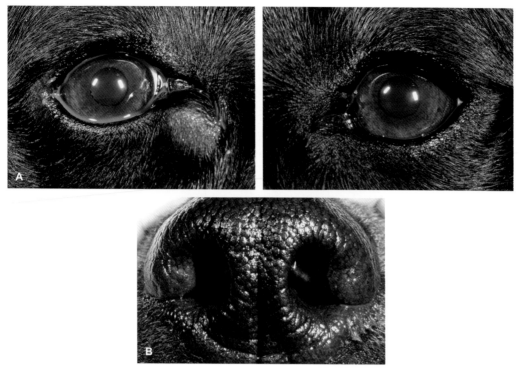

Fig. 4.1c (A) Both eyes following the application of fluorescein dye. Accumulation of fluorescein within the meniscus of the tear film and overflow at the medial canthus suggest abnormal nasolacrimal drainage in the right eye. (B) Fluorescein dye is only visible at the left nares (positive Jones test).

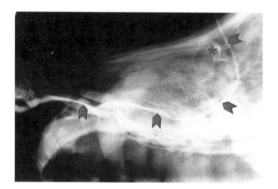

Fig. 4.1d Dacryocystorhinogram showing contrast material filling the duct (arrows). Spillage of contrast material is present on the eyelid skin and around the nostril (asterix). Reproduced with permission from RN White.

The plain radiographs in this dog are normal. The lateral dacryocystorhinogram demonstrates contrast material evenly filling the length of the nasolacrimal duct from the eye to the distal nasal ostium. The duct appears normal with respect to its course and diameter (Fig. 4.1d).
- CT scan – this is performed to evaluate the nature of the swelling at the ventromedial canthus and to determine whether it is associated with the nasolacrimal duct.

In this dog, the swelling is cystic and compresses the proximal part of the nasolacrimal duct; contrast material fills the entire length of the nasolacrimal duct and there is no physical connection with the lumen of the cyst (Fig. 4.1e).

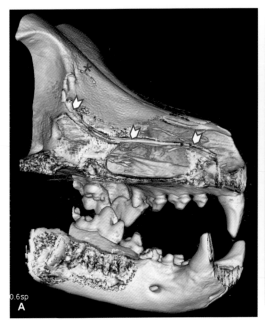 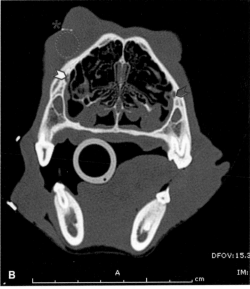

Fig. 4.1e CT scans. (A) 3-D volume rendered image of the skull, with the lateral surface of the incisive and maxillary bones removed. Contrast material fills the length of the normal nasolacrimal duct (arrows). (B) Transverse scan at the level of the cyst. Contrast material is visible within the right nasolacrimal duct (white arrow) but not within the cyst (dotted circle). The left nasolacrimal duct does not contain contrast material (red arrow). There is a small amount of skin contamination by contrast material (asterix).

Diagnosis

Based on the information available, the diagnosis is compression of the right nasolacrimal duct by a cyst.

Treatment

Surgical excision of the cyst is indicated because, if left untreated, it is likely to enlarge. Under general anaesthesia, the nasolacrimal duct is cannulated with blue 2/0 nylon suture material. The coloured suture material highlights the position of the duct and minimises the risk of inadvertent damage. The cyst is carefully dissected from the surrounding tissue and totally excised; the soft tissues are closed routinely. The nasolacrimal duct is flushed in a normograde direction to confirm patency. Postoperative medication includes systemic broad-spectrum antibiotic and NSAID therapy for five days.

Prognosis

The prognosis for the resolution of epiphora in the right eye is excellent if the nasolacrimal duct is not damaged and if the cyst lining is entirely removed.

Discussion

Cysts of the nasolacrimal system and associated structures are uncommon and are generally presumed to be congenital. A thorough investigation is indicated to establish whether the cyst has a physical connection with the nasolacrimal system and in order to facilitate accurate surgical planning. If there is a connection (dacryops or canaliculops), even meticulous surgery can cause damage and permanent obstruction to the nasolacrimal system. Excellent illumination, magnification and microinstrumentation are essential requirements for successful surgery of the nasolacrimal system.

Further reading

See Appendix 2.

History

A four-year-old male neutered domestic shorthaired cat is presented with a three-week history of a thick discharge from the left eye which is unresponsive to topical fusidic acid and gentamicin. The owner has also noticed that the cat has been grooming the left side of its face more frequently than usual. The cat has received routine vaccinations and anthelmintic treatment; he is an indoor/outdoor cat and is otherwise well.

Questions

1. Describe the abnormalities and pertinent normal features in Figs. 4.2a and b.
2. What differential diagnoses should be considered for this presentation?
3. What tests could you perform to make the diagnosis?

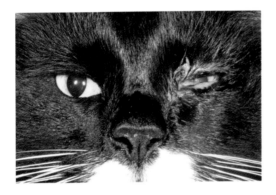

Fig. 4.2a

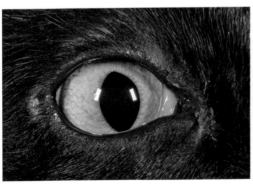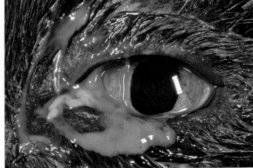

Fig. 4.2b

Answers

1. What the figures show
Fig. 4.2a The right eye is normal. Left eye – the palpebral fissure is narrowed and there is a marked mucopurulent ocular discharge.

Fig. 4.2b Left eye – there is a small amount of caseous material at the medial canthus in addition to copious mucopurulent discharge on the eyelids and periocular hair. The lustrous ocular surface and normal Purkinje image are consistent with a good tear film.

2. Differential diagnoses
Given the appearance of the left eye, the clinical diagnosis is mucopurulent ocular discharge for which the following conditions should be considered:

- **Dacryocystitis** Inflammation of the nasolacrimal sac in the cat is most commonly associated with feline herpesvirus-1 (FHV-1) infection. It can lead to the formation of a stricture within the duct and permanent epiphora. Dacryocystitis can also be caused by a primary bacterial infection or a foreign body lodged in the nasolacrimal sac or duct. Clinical signs include epiphora, purulent ocular discharge, conjunctivitis, discomfort and occasionally, a draining skin fistula ventral to the medial canthus.
- **Infectious conjunctivitis** This is very common in the cat, the two most important causes being FHV-1 and *Chlamydophila felis* (*C felis*) (*Ch. 6, case 1*). The ocular discharge is generally serous and represents increased lacrimation caused by conjunctivitis and ocular irritation. The discharge may become mucoid or mucopurulent with secondary bacterial involvement, most commonly by *Staphylococcus* sp or other Gram-positive organisms. A foreign body in the conjunctival fornices, behind the TEL or within the nasolacrimal sac and duct can cause secondary bacterial conjunctivitis.
- **Keratoconjunctivitis sicca (KCS)** KCS is characterised by a deficiency of the aqueous component of the tear film and is uncommon in the cat. Feline KCS is usually associated with blepharoconjunctivitis, as opposed to immune-mediated KCS in the dog. A tenacious mucoid or mucopurulent ocular discharge is the hallmark of canine KCS but clinical signs in the cat are often subtle. The diagnosis of KCS in the cat is usually based on the combination of low tear production and compatible clinical signs, although Schirmer test values are highly variable in the cat.
- **Qualitative tear film deficiency** This is characterised by an abnormality of the lipid or mucin layers of the tear film and is uncommon in both cats and dogs. Although a mucoid discharge is typically present in affected dogs, cats usually present with ulcerative keratitis, acceptable aqueous tear production and a rapid tear film break-up time.

Tear film break-up time (TBUT) is a measure of the stability of the tear film, as measured by the time taken for the tear film to dissociate from the ocular surface. Fluorescein dye is applied to the ocular surface, the eye is allowed to blink and then the eyelids are held open. The time it takes for the first dark spot to appear in the tear film is measured. This procedure is facilitated by slit-lamp biomicroscopy and a cobalt-blue filter. The average TBUT is 20 s in the dog and 16.7 s in the cat.

3. Appropriate diagnostic tests
- Ocular reflexes
  - Pupillary light reflex – direct and consensual positive OU
  - Dazzle reflex – positive OU
  - Palpebral reflex – positive OU

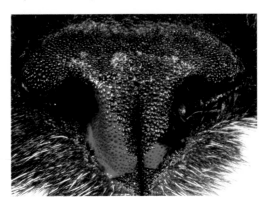

Fig. 4.2c Jones test: right side positive, left side negative. Note the small amount of fluorescein dye below the left nares which has spread from the right nostril.

- Menace response – positive OU
- Examination with a focal light source – the ocular discharge is removed from the left eye. There is marked hyperaemia of the palpebral, bulbar and TEL conjunctiva. Magnification is helpful to evaluate the nasolacrimal puncta but even with slit-lamp biomicroscopy the puncta are difficult to discern because of the conjunctival swelling.
- Schirmer tear test – 16 mm/min OS, 19 mm/min OD
- Fluorescein dye
  - Staining – negative OU
  - Jones test (fluorescein dye passage test) – positive OD, negative OS. This is suggestive of reduced tear drainage in the left eye (Fig. 4.2c).
- Tonometry – IOP 17 mmHg OU
- Cytology (ocular discharge) – this reveals a large population of neutrophils, some of which contain cocci.
- Culture (ocular discharge) – this reveals a heavy mixed growth of *Staphylococcus aureus* and *Escherichia coli*.

A more detailed examination is performed whilst the cat is under general anaesthesia and reveals a focal swelling ventral to the medial canthus of the left eye. The remainder of the ophthalmic examination reveals no additional abnormalities and a general physical examination is unremarkable.

Further diagnostic tests
- Nasolacrimal duct cannulation and flush (performed under general anaesthesia) – flushing in a normograde direction (eye to nose) results in the expression of a copious amount of mucupurulent material from both puncta but no fluid from the ipsilateral nostril. These findings are consistent with a nasolacrimal duct obstruction (Fig. 4.2d).

Cannulation of the nasolacrimal punctum can be performed with a metal or plastic lacrimal cannula. The size of the cannula (22–25 gauge) depends on the size of the animal; plastic cannulas with an outer diameter of 0.9 mm in the dog and 0.76 mm in the cat are usually appropriate. Cutting the plastic cannula short and at an oblique angle facilitates cannulation. Intravenous catheters (with the metal stylet removed) can also be used. Sterile saline is usually used for flushing although tap water, distilled water and lactated Ringer's solution are acceptable alternatives. Cannulation of the upper punctum is generally preferred because it avoids the risk of inadvertent damage to the lower punctum which is responsible for the majority of tear drainage, and because it is usually easier.

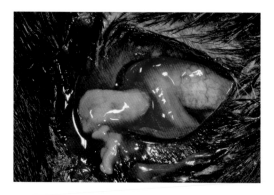

Fig. 4.2d Copious mucopurulent discharge and caseous material are expressed from the puncta during flushing of the nasolacrimal duct.

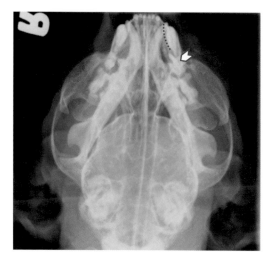

Fig. 4.2e Dorsoventral dacryocystorhinogram. There is contrast material within the proximal nasolacrimal duct (arrow) up to the level of the root of the maxillary canine tooth; the dotted line indicates the course of the nasolacrimal duct to the distal nasal ostium.

- Radiography – radiographic evaluation of the nasolacrimal system requires plain radiography followed by a contrast study (dacryocystorhinography). Following cannulation, radiopaque contrast material is injected into the upper punctum until it emerges from the ipsilateral nostril (0.5 ml in a cat).

  In this cat, the plain radiographs are normal. The dorsoventral dacryocystorhinogram demonstrates contrast material within the proximal region of the duct (arrow) which stops at the level of the root of the maxillary canine tooth (Fig. 4.2e).

Diagnosis

Based on the information available, a diagnosis of dacryocystitis and proximal obstruction of the nasolacrimal duct in the left eye is made.

Treatment

Surgical exploration of the proximal nasolacrimal duct is indicated because of the poor response to medical management. The upper and lower puncta are both cannulated with a plastic cannula; the cannula tips are advanced until they contact each other within the lacrimal sac (Allgoewer and Nöller, 2009, Fig. 4.2f, A). An incision is made in the conjunctiva overlying the lacrimal sac and a second incision through the skin overlying the swelling ventral to the medial canthus. The lacrimal sac is explored by blunt dissection (Fig. 4.2f, B) and a grass seed foreign body is discovered and

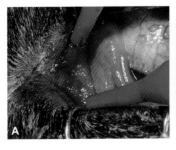
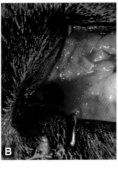
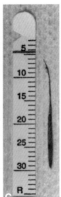
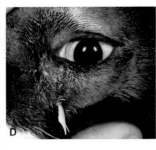

Fig. 4.2f (A) Placement of a plastic nasolacrimal cannula (outer diameter 0.76 mm) in each of the upper and lower punctum. (B) Exploration of the lacrimal sac. (C) Identification and removal of a grass seed foreign body. (D) Routine closure incorporating a mini Penrose drain.

removed (Fig. 4.2f, C). The lacrimal sac is irrigated with saline and the soft tissues are closed routinely. A mini Penrose drain is inserted (Fig. 4.2f, D) and removed after 48 hours. Systemic broad-spectrum antibiotic and NSAID therapy is continued for a week.

Prognosis
The short-term prognosis for resolution of the ocular discharge is excellent. However, because of the severity of the dacryocystitis and the potential for stricture formation within the nasolacrimal duct, permanent epiphora is a likely complication in this cat.

Discussion
Severe unilateral mucopurulent ocular discharge is an uncommon clinical presentation in the cat and each case should be approached in a systematic manner in order to reach an accurate diagnosis and instigate appropriate management. Appropriate illumination and magnification as well as microinstrumentation are essential requirements for successful surgery of the nasolacrimal system.

Further reading
Allgoewer I & Nöller C (2009) A surgical technique for dacryocystotomy in dogs with foreign body induced dacryocystitis. *Proc Eur Coll Vet Ophthalmol, Copenhagen 2009, Vet Ophthal*, **12** (6), 379–389.

See Appendix 2.

History

A seven-year-old female neutered cross-breed dog is presented with a four-week history of a thick green discharge from the left eye which has been unresponsive to topical fusidic acid. The dog has received routine vaccinations and anthelmintic treatment and is otherwise clinically well.

Questions

1. Describe the abnormalities and pertinent normal features in Figs. 4.3a, b and c.
2. What differential diagnoses should be considered for this presentation?
3. What tests could you perform to make the diagnosis?

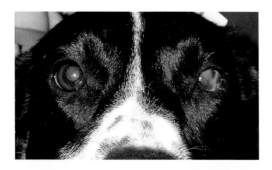

Fig. 4.3a

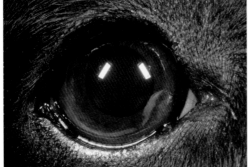

Fig. 4.3b

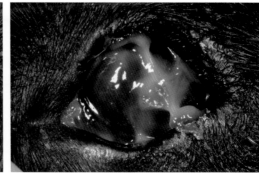

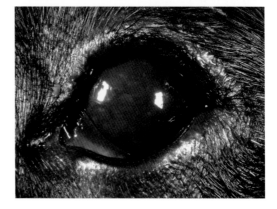

Fig. 4.3c

Answers

1. What the figures show
Fig. 4.3a The right eye is normal. Left eye – the palpebral fissure is slightly narrowed and there is a marked mucopurulent ocular discharge.

Fig. 4.3b Left eye – there is a slight protrusion of the TEL. A tenacious mucopurulent discharge is adherent to the ocular surface. The Purkinje images are disrupted.

Fig. 4.3c The left eye after the discharge has been flushed from the ocular surface. There is generalised corneal pigmentation which prevents assessment of intraocular structures.

2. Differential diagnoses
Given the appearance of the left eye, the clinical diagnosis is mucopurulent discharge for which the following conditions should be considered:

- **Keratoconjunctivitis sicca (KCS)** A common ocular condition in the dog which results from a deficiency in the aqueous component of the tear film. There is desiccation of the ocular surface, discomfort, and reduced vision. Clinical signs of early KCS include a mucoid or mucopurulent discharge and conjunctivitis which can be misdiagnosed as a primary bacterial conjunctivitis. The hallmark of KCS is that the ocular discharge is tenacious and adheres to the ocular surface. This is in contrast to ocular discharge that is readily removed from the ocular surface during blinking in eyes with an adequate tear film. With more advanced disease, there is a lack-lustre appearance to the ocular surface. The most common form of KCS in the dog is a bilateral, tissue-specific, immune-mediated disorder. Other causes of bilateral disease include viral adenitis (canine distemper virus), drug induced (systemic sulphonamides, etodolac, and atropine), and endocrine disease (diabetes mellitus, hypothyroidism, and hyperadrenocorticism). Unilateral disease is less common but can result from congenital lacrimal gland aplasia/hypoplasia, topical atropine, excision of the TEL gland, uncorrected prolapse of the TEL gland, neurotrophic keratitis (loss of sensation to the ocular surface), neurologic deficits (loss of parasympathetic innervation to the lacrimal gland), orbital disease, local radiation therapy and chronic blepharoconjunctivitis.

- **Qualitative tear film deficiency** This refers to an abnormality of the lipid or mucin components of the tear film. The deficiency is usually bilateral. The majority of cases in the dog are associated with abnormalities of the eyelid margin (e.g. meibomianitis, chalazia, generalised skin disease) and other clinical signs include ocular discomfort, mucoid discharge, conjunctivitis, superficial keratitis, tear film instability (rapid TBUT), and corneal ulceration (*Ch. 2, case 3*). The diagnosis of qualitative tear film disorders can be challenging but ocular surface disease in the presence of normal aqueous tear production (i.e. a normal STT value) and the absence of other identifiable causes should increase the index of suspicion.

> Tear film break-up time (TBUT) is a measure of the stability of the tear film. TBUT is a measure of the time taken for the tear film to dissociate from the ocular surface. Fluorescein dye is applied to the ocular surface, the eye is allowed to blink and then the eyelids are held open. The time is takes for the first dark spot to appear in the tear film is measured. This procedure is facilitated by slit-lamp biomicroscopy and a cobalt-blue filter. The average TBUT is 20 s in the dog and 16.7 s in the cat.

- **Bacterial conjunctivitis** Secondary bacterial conjunctivitis is common in the dog. The clinical presentation can be unilateral or bilateral and signs include a mucopurulent ocular discharge in the presence of normal or increased tear production. The discharge accumulates along the eyelid margins and at the medial canthus as it is removed from the ocular surface during blinking, in contrast to the tenacious discharge in KCS. Causes of bacterial conjunctivitis include an eyelid mass, eyelid irregularity and a foreign body (behind the TEL, in the conjunctival fornices or in the nasolacrimal sac/duct). Bacterial conjunctivitis can occur secondary to KCS because of the loss of immunoprotective properties in the aqueous component of the tear film. Primary bacterial conjunctivitis is uncommon in dogs; the most common organisms are *Staphylococcus* sp and other Gram-positive organisms.

- **Dacryocystitis** Inflammation of the nasolacrimal sac is a common condition in the dog and is usually caused by a foreign body lodged in the nasolacrimal sac or duct. Clinical signs include epiphora, purulent discharge, conjunctivitis, discomfort and occasionally a draining skin fistula ventral to the medial canthus.
- **Canine distemper virus (CDV)** Ocular manifestations of CDV include conjunctivitis, KCS, chorioretinitis and optic neuritis. A mucopurulent ocular discharge is usually associated with the conjunctivitis that occurs during the initial episode of pyrexia, rhinitis and tracheobronchitis.

3. Appropriate diagnostic tests
- Ocular reflexes
  - Pupillary light reflex – the left pupil is not visible. Positive consensual OS (from left to right eye); positive direct OD.
  - Dazzle reflex – positive OU
  - Palpebral reflex – positive OU
  - Corneal reflex – positive OU

Corneal sensation can be assessed by touching a wisp of cotton wool to the lateral region of the cornea (i.e. away from the visual axis); if a blink response is elicited, corneal sensation is said to be present. Corneal sensation can be semi-quantified with a corneal aesthesiometer, e.g. a Cochet-Bonnet or Larson-Millodot aesthesiometer. This instrument consists of a fine filament, which is adjustable in length – the filament is touched to the cornea to elicit a blink. The length of filament required to elicit a blink determines the corneal touch threshold (CTT). CTT is determined in different regions of the cornea. Skull shape influences corneal sensitivity in dogs and cats – the cornea in brachycephalic dogs and cats is less sensitive than in dolichocephalic dog breeds and non-brachycephalic cats.

- Vision assessment
  - Menace response – positive OU
  - Tracking reflex – equivocal OS and positive OD
  - Maze test (obstacle course) – the dog can navigate around large objects in both photopic and scotopic conditions.

In this dog, these findings are consistent with reduced vision in the left eye.

- Examination with a focal light source – in the left eye, this reveals hyperaemia and hyperpigmentation of the palpebral conjunctivae, generalised corneal pigmentation, and an anterior chamber of normal depth. Superficial corneal vascularisation is seen with slit-lamp biomicroscopy.
- Ophthalmoscopy – this is not possible in the left eye because of the corneal pigmentation. Fundic examination in the right eye is unremarkable.

- Schirmer tear test – 0 mm/min OS, 19 mm/min OD. This is consistent with absent tear production in the left eye.
- Fluorescein dye
  - Staining – diffuse positive 'stippling' OS, negative OD. This is consistent with poor ocular surface health in the left eye.
  - Jones test (fluorescein dye passage test) – negative OS, positive OD. This is consistent with reduced tear drainage in the left eye.
  - Tear film break-up time – 5 s OS, 20 s OD. This is consistent with poor tear film stability in the left eye.
- Tonometry – IOP 17 mmHg OU
- Cytology (ocular discharge) – this reveals a large population of neutrophils, some of which contain cocci.
- Culture (ocular discharge) – this reveals a heavy mixed growth of *Staphylococcus aureus* and *Bacillus* sp.

Following topical anaesthesia, the posterior aspect of the TEL is examined for the presence of a foreign body and none is found. The remainder of the ophthalmic examination reveals no additional abnormalities. A general physical examination reveals left-side xeromycteria (nasal dryness) (Fig. 4.3d) and a notable absence of xerostomia (dry oral mucous membranes).

Further diagnostic tests
- Nasolacrimal duct cannulation and flush (following topical anaesthesia) – flushing in a normograde direction (eye to nose) results in saline appearing at the ipsilateral nostril. This confirms that the nasolacrimal duct is patent and that the negative Jones test is because of reduced tear drainage caused by the thick mucopurulent discharge within the nasolacrimal system.

Cannulation of the nasolacrimal punctum can be performed with a metal or plastic lacrimal cannula. The size of the cannula (22–25 gauge) depends on the size of the animal; plastic cannulas with an outer diameter of 0.9 mm in the dog and 0.76 mm in the cat are usually appropriate. Cutting the plastic cannula short and at an oblique angle facilitates cannulation. Intravenous catheters (with the metal stylet removed) can also be used. Sterile saline is usually used for flushing although tap water, distilled water and lactated Ringer's solution are acceptable alternatives. Cannulation of the upper punctum is generally preferred because it avoids the risk of inadvertent damage to the lower punctum which is responsible for the majority of tear drainage, and because it is usually easier.

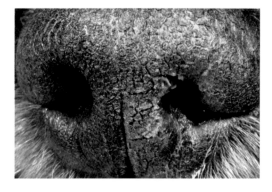

Fig. 4.3d Left-sided xeromycteria.

- Radiography – plain skull radiography to evaluate the tympanic bullae and the region of the petrous temporal bone is unremarkable.

Diagnosis

Based on the information available, a diagnosis of neurogenic KCS in the left eye is made. Unilateral KCS with ipsilateral xeromycteria is considered pathognomonic for neurogenic KCS. The most likely location of the neurologic deficit is the middle and/or inner ear.

Treatment

Neurogenic KCS can be frustrating to manage but medical and surgical management options are available. Medical treatment includes topical tear replacement therapy and the direct stimulation of tear production (lacrimostimulant drugs). The aim of tear replacement therapy is to provide lubrication of the ocular surface in order to alleviate ocular discomfort and minimise progressive corneal pathology. Numerous tear replacement products are available and the specific selection depends primarily on the duration of action required. Owner compliance is usually improved by minimising the frequency of topical treatments. For this reason, a long-acting product is indicated in this dog as the tear production is zero in the affected eye, e.g. carbomer polymer gel, hyaluronic acid or paraffin-based ointment. Lacrimostimulants include both immunomodulatory drugs and parasympathomimetic agents. Topical cyclosporine is the only licensed immunomodulatory drug in the dog and is indicated for immune-mediated KCS. Parasympathomimetic agents are more likely to be useful for neurogenic KCS because lacrimal gland secretion is principally controlled by parasympathetic fibres (carried by the facial nerve). Pilocarpine is a direct-acting parasympathomimetic drug which is generally used orally because the topical form is irritant and is often less effective than oral administration.

The majority of cases of neurogenic KCS are idiopathic although involvement of the middle/inner ear is implicated. Some dogs respond to prolonged systemic broad-spectrum antibiotic and NSAID therapy, which are used on the basis of a presumptive inflammatory/infectious process.

Unfortunately, this dog is unresponsive to an intensive medical regime comprising tear replacement therapy, systemic pilocarpine and a six-week course of clavulanate-potentiated amoxicillin and carprofen. Surgical management in the form of a parotid duct transposition (PDT) is elected because of the failure of medical treatment. The function of the parotid gland and duct is confirmed prior to surgery by the application of lemon juice to the dog's tongue followed by direct observation of the parotid papilla for signs of secretion. An open (lateral) approach is chosen for the PDT.

The parotid duct conducts saliva from the parotid gland to an oral papilla near the carnassial tooth (parotid papilla). In a PDT, the duct and papilla are mobilised and translocated to the lower conjunctival sac to provide moisture for the ocular surface. A PDT is indicated for cases of KCS that are unresponsive to medical management. Two surgical approaches are described: an 'open' approach which is performed through a lateral facial skin incision, and a 'closed' approach performed through an oral incision.

Lemon juice is bitter and stimulates salivation (sialogogue). Although atropine is a parasympatholytic agent which reduces salivation, it is also bitter and is widely used by veterinary ophthalmologists as a sialogogue prior to PDT surgery.

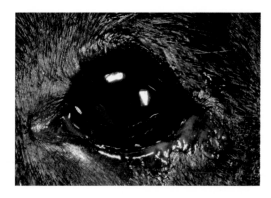

Fig. 4.3e Left eye 24 hours after PDT surgery. The ocular surface appears moist and lustrous – there is a meniscus of saliva along the eyelid margins and the Purkinje images are normal. Note the salivary secretion spilling over the edge of the lower eyelid.

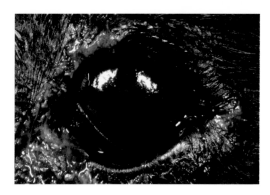

Fig. 4.3f Left eye six months after PDT surgery. The tenacious mucopurulent ocular discharge has resolved and the ocular surface appears moist. There is mineral deposition on the eyelids and the cornea, and the latter causes disruption of the Purkinje images.

Although the ocular surface of the left eye is moist and lustrous immediately following surgery (Fig. 4.3e), saliva contains a higher concentration of minerals than the tear film and mineral deposition can be seen on the cornea, eyelid margin and periocular skin six months after surgery (Fig. 4.3f).

The ocular surface flora also changes significantly following a PDT and may consist of large numbers of a mixed population of bacteria, uncommon isolates and potential pathogens – this can contribute to chronic blepharitis following surgery.

Following surgery, this dog is managed long-term with daily cleansing of the eye and periocular skin with water, intermittent use of a barrier cream on the periocular skin (paraffin-based ophthalmic ointment) and topical and systemic broad-spectrum antibiotics to address recurrent, secondary bacterial infections.

Prognosis

The prognosis for the control of neurogenic KCS is guarded because most dogs are unresponsive to medical treatment, and in the few that do respond, long-term treatment is usually indicated. The prognosis for a comfortable, visual eye with stable corneal disease following PDT surgery is fair to good. However, complications are common and include transient subcutaneous oedema, sialolith formation, and blepharoconjunctivitis and discomfort because of mineral deposition on the ocular surface and eyelids. Transection or twisting of the duct at the time of surgery can lead to stricture formation and obstruction to the flow of saliva. Owners must be aware that some level of long-term maintenance is required in almost all dogs that have undergone PDT.

Discussion

Neurologic disease is an uncommon cause of KCS in the dog but it is important to recognise its characteristic clinical presentation so that the appropriate treatment and prognosis can be given. Neurogenic KCS is most often acute in onset, unilateral and accompanied by ipsilateral xeromycteria. This is quite different from the gradual onset, bilateral nature of immune-mediated KCS which is typical of predisposed breeds such as the West Highland White Terrier. The xeromycteria is because of denervation of the parasympathetic supply to the lateral nasal gland located within the distal nasal cavity, rather than a result of the thick ocular discharge.

Further reading

See Appendix 2.

CHAPTER 5

The Painful Eye

Introduction

It can be difficult to recognise that an eye is painful, but increased lacrimation, photophobia, and particularly blepharospasm are strong indicators, regardless of whether the pain originates from the ocular surface or from intraocular disease. Owners are more likely to notice a change in the appearance of the eye than to recognise that a closed eye is an indication of pain.

Small Animal Ophthalmology: What's Your Diagnosis? First Edition. Heidi Featherstone, Elaine Holt.
© 2011 by Heidi Featherstone and Elaine Holt. Published 2011 by Blackwell Publishing Ltd.

History

A one-year-old female neutered Flat-Coated Retriever is presented with a 24-hour history of a painful, wet right eye. The dog has received routine vaccinations and anthelmintic treatment and is otherwise well.

Questions

1. Describe the abnormalities and pertinent normal features in Fig. 5.1a.
2. What differential diagnoses should be considered for this presentation?
3. What tests could you perform to make the diagnosis?

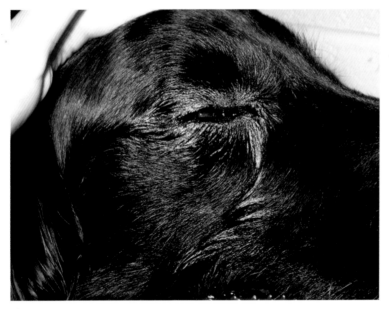

Fig. 5.1a

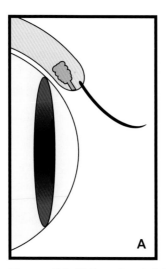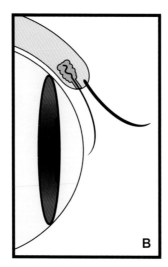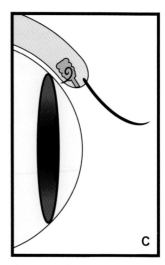

Diagram 5.1 (A) Normal eyelash (B) Distichium (C) Ectopic cilium. Illustration by S Scurrell.

Answers

1. What the figure shows

Fig. 5.1a Right eye – there is marked epiphora and periocular wetting. The palpebral fissure is almost closed.

2. Differential diagnoses

Given the history and the appearance of the right eye, the clinical diagnosis is excessive lacrimation, for which the following conditions should be considered:

- **Ectopic cilia** This is a condition in which extra eyelashes arise from the region of the meibomian glands but, in contrast to distichiasis, emerge through the palpebral conjunctiva 4–6 mm from the eyelid margin. Ectopic cilia most commonly occur in the centre of the upper eyelid and cause direct irritation to the ocular surface (Diagram 5.1). The typical clinical presentation is acute onset blepharospasm, lacrimation and corneal ulceration in a young dog (usually less than one year old). Clinical signs may be intermittent because ectopic cilia eventually fall out, only to regrow several weeks later. Predisposed breeds include the Lhasa Apso, Pekingese, Shih Tzu, Poodle, English Bulldog, Flat-Coated Retriever and Boxer.
- **Distichiasis** This is a common condition in which extra eyelashes arise from the region of the meibomian glands and emerge from, or just posterior to, the gland openings along the eyelid margin (Diagram 5.1). Distichiasis tends to occur in dogs less than one year old. It is often an incidental finding, but it can cause increased lacrimation, epiphora, and blepharospasm; corneal ulceration is uncommon. The degree of corneal irritation is related to the number, length and direction of the distichia. Short, stiff distichia tend to cause irritation whereas long, soft distichia cause little if any irritation unless they are present in high numbers and/or are directed towards the ocular surface. Distichia may act as a wick, causing tears to overflow onto the periocular hairs, mimicking a problem with tear drainage. Predisposed breeds are the Cocker Spaniel (American and English), Boxer, English Bulldog, Flat-Coated Retriever, Shih Tzu, Pekingese, Poodle, Dachsund and Jack Russell Terrier (*Ch. 2, case 2*).
- **Entropion** This refers to the inversion or inward turning of part or all of the eyelid margin. Hair consequently contacts the ocular surface (trichiasis) and causes pain because of associated

conjunctivitis, keratitis and/or corneal ulceration. Entropion can involve different regions of the eyelid but lower lateral entropion is frequently encountered in clinical practice (*Ch. 2, case 1*).

- **Corneal ulcer** With the exception of neurotrophic ulcerative keratitis (*Ch. 12, case 1*), corneal ulcers are invariably associated with mild to severe ocular discomfort. Superficial ulcers are usually more painful than deep ulcers, because the anterior corneal stroma has a high proportion of pain receptors, whereas the deep corneal stroma is rich in pressure receptors.
- **Trauma/foreign body** Blunt or penetrating trauma, and corneal or conjunctival foreign bodies can cause ocular pain and excessive lacrimation. Trauma usually results in acute, unilateral ocular signs (*Ch. 12*).
- **Eyelid swellings** Any irregularity of the normal contour of the eyelid margin has the potential to cause ocular discomfort, e.g. chalazion (*Ch. 2, case 3*), hordoleum (stye), granuloma, neoplasia, and blepharitis.
- **Trichiasis** This is a condition in which periocular hairs growing in a normal location are abnormally directed towards the ocular surface. If severe, trichiasis can cause conjunctivitis and keratitis, with associated discomfort. Trichiasis results from entropion and eyelid agenesis and can also be associated with the nasal folds, medial canthus and caruncle.
- **Anterior uveitis** Pain as a result of spasm of the iris sphincter and ciliary body muscles occurs with anterior uveitis, often referred to 'brow ache' in humans. There is also usually some degree of blepharospasm and increased lacrimation (*Ch. 7, case 3*).
- **Glaucoma** Pain as a result of stimulation of the pressure and stretch receptors is most marked in acute rather than chronic glaucoma and dogs frequently show increased lacrimation, photophobia, and head-shy behaviour (*Ch. 6, case 2*).
- **Eyelid agenesis or coloboma** Localised absence of eyelid tissue results in increased exposure of the ocular surface, trichiasis and a reduced ability to blink; together these cause conjunctivitis and keratitis, with associated discomfort. Eyelid agenesis is most common in the lateral upper eyelid of cats; it is rarely seen in the dog.

3. Appropriate diagnostic tests

The right eye is so painful that the dog is unable to open it. Examination is facilitated by the use of topical anaesthesia which quickly alleviates the blepharospasm (Fig. 5.1b, A).

A single drop of a topical anaesthetic drug will anaesthetise the ocular surface (conjunctiva and cornea) within approximately 10 s. Anaesthesia lasts for about 45 min in the normal dog eye (25 min in the cat). The depth and duration of anaesthesia can be increased by repeat application of the topical anaesthetic, e.g. one drop applied twice over one min. The application of a topical anaesthetic can be a simple way of differentiating surface ocular pain from pain caused by intraocular or orbital disease.

- Ocular reflexes
  - Pupillary light reflex – direct and consensual positive OU
  - Dazzle reflex – positive OU
  - Palpebral reflex – positive OU
- Menace response – positive OU
- Examination with a focal light source – this reveals several fine hairs along the eyelid margins and protrusion of the TEL in both eyes. There is a grey gelatinous discharge in the lower conjunctival fornix of the left eye (arrow) (Fig. 5.1b, B), and a relative anisocoria (OD < OS). With slit-lamp biomicroscopy a single pigmented hair is visible emerging from the palpebral conjunc-

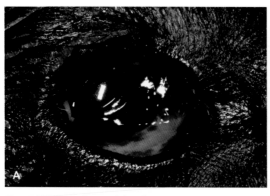
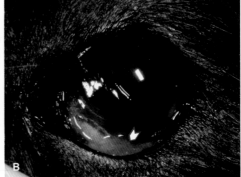

Fig. 5.1b (A) Right eye (B) Left eye

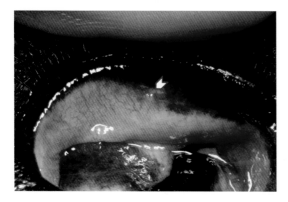

Fig. 5.1c The right upper eyelid is manually everted to reveal a single pigmented ectopic cilium (arrow) emerging from the palpebral conjunctiva.

tival surface; the hair is posterior to the line of the meibomian gland openings and in the centre of the upper eyelid of the right eye (arrow, Fig. 5.1c).

- Schirmer tear test – 17 mm/min OS. This test is not performed OD because of the excessive lacrimation.
- Fluorescein dye
  ○ Staining – negative OS, positive 'stippling' in the dorsal and ventromedial region of the cornea OD. This is suggestive of minor physical disruption to the tear film in the right eye.
  ○ Jones test (fluorescein dye passage test) – positive OU
- Tonometry – IOP 17 mmHg OU

The posterior aspect of the TEL is examined for the presence of a foreign body and none is found. The remainder of the ophthalmic examination reveals no additional abnormalities and a general physical examination is unremarkable.

Diagnosis

Based on the information available, a diagnosis of an ectopic cilium in the right eye and distichiasis in both eyes is made.

The relative miosis in the right eye is because of reflex uveitis. Corneal stimulation incites an axonal reflex mediated by substance P and results in iridocyclospasm and subsequent miosis (*Ch. 10, case 1*). Enophthalmos and TEL protrusion can also be a direct response to ocular pain. When unilateral ocular pain is marked, it is not uncommon to see bilateral protrusion of the TEL. The distichiasis in both eyes is considered to be incidental given that the ocular pain and excessive lacrimation are unilateral. The grey gelatinous discharge noted in the left eye is a common feature of dog breeds with deep orbits, narrow skull conformation and poor tear drainage. Referred to as 'medial canthal pocket syndrome', it can cause mild but chronic conjunctivitis. Predisposed breeds include the Doberman Pinscher, Great Dane, Standard Poodle, Afghan Hound, Weimaraner and Flat-Coated Retriever.

Treatment

Ectopic cilia must be treated surgically. Treatment involves excision of the ectopic cilium/cilia and its hair follicle; other options include destruction of the hair follicle by electrocautery or cryosurgery. In this dog, under general anaesthesia, and with the aid of an operating microscope, the upper eyelid is stabilised within a Desmarres chalazion clamp – the ectopic cilium and surrounding conjunctiva are then excised *en bloc* using a 2-mm biopsy punch (Fig. 5.1d). The conjunctival wound is left to heal by secondary intention. Further examination reveals a second pigmented ectopic cilium on the posterior aspect of the TEL which is also excised *en bloc* (Fig. 5.1e). Postoperative medication comprises topical broad-spectrum antibiotic and systemic NSAID therapy for three days.

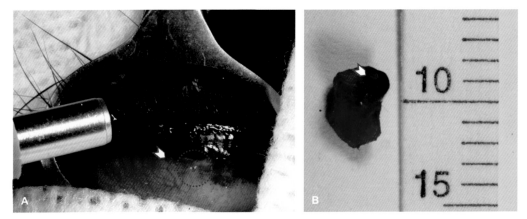

Fig. 5.1d (A) Area of tissue to be excised by 2-mm biopsy punch. (B) Excised conjunctiva containing ectopic cilium (arrow) and its follicle.

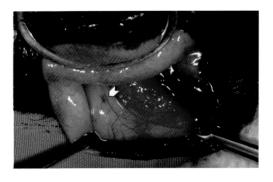

Fig. 5.1e Pigmented leading edge of the TEL is retracted to reveal a pigmented ectopic cilium emerging from the conjunctiva on the posterior surface (arrow).

Prognosis

The prognosis for the resolution of the ocular discomfort and excessive lacrimation is excellent following excision of ectopic cilia. Recurrence is unlikely if the hair follicle is completely excised but additional cilia may emerge from adjacent sites. In general, dogs affected with ectopic cilia are also predisposed to distichiasis and *vice versa*. The risk of developing either condition appears to diminish with increasing age.

Discussion

The typical clinical presentation for ectopic cilia is acute onset, unilateral ocular discomfort in a young dog for which no other obvious cause can be identified. Ectopic cilia most frequently arise from the centre of the upper eyelid and appear as single or multiple hairs. The colour of the ectopic cilia usually correlates to coat colour and the diagnosis is therefore especially challenging in lightly coloured breeds because the ectopic cilia may be non-pigmented, e.g. English Bulldog.

A corneal ulcer may develop and its location will correspond to the position of the ectopic cilia. The hallmark of a corneal ulcer secondary to ectopic cilia is its slightly dorsal location and a vertical elliptical shape – the latter is caused by the vertical direction of eyelid movement. Ectopic cilia which arise from the posterior aspect of the TEL are uncommon, however this dog demonstrates that ectopic cilia can be multiple and arise in any location. The diagnosis of ectopic cilia is challenging without good magnification (slit-lamp biomicroscope and/or an operating microscope) but the clinical presentation should always raise a high index of suspicion.

Further reading

See Appendix 2.

CASE STUDY 2

History
A five-year-old male neutered British shorthaired cat is presented with a 24-hour history of a painful and wet left eye. The cat has a previous history of ulcerative keratitis in the right eye. He lives in a multi-cat household; all the cats have received routine vaccinations and anthelmintic treatment, and are indoor/outdoor cats. None of the cats has been in a cattery or has a history of upper respiratory tract infection.

Questions
1. Describe the abnormalities and pertinent normal features in Figs. 5.2a and b.
2. What differential diagnoses should be considered for this presentation?
3. What tests could you perform to make the diagnosis?

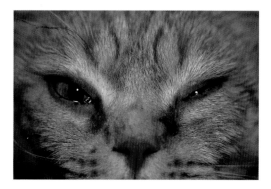

Fig. 5.2a

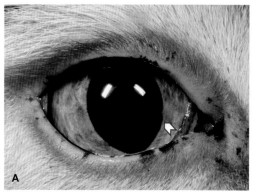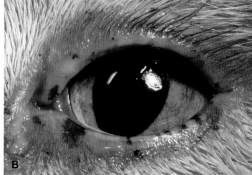

Fig. 5.2b

Answers

1. What the figures show
Fig. 5.2a Left eye – there is epiphora and dark tear staining at the medial canthus. The palpebral fissure is narrow. The right eye appears normal.

Fig. 5.2b Left eye – the periocular region is wet and the Purkinje images are disrupted. Right eye – there is a subtle, poorly defined corneal opacity (arrow). The Purkinje images are normal.

2. Differential diagnoses
Given the history and the appearance of the left eye, the following conditions should be considered:

- **Qualitative tear film disorder** This refers to an abnormality of the mucin or lipid components of the tear film. An association between ulcerative keratitis and a deficiency of mucin has been described in the cat (Cullen *et al.*, 1999). The condition is usually bilateral and often characterised by the development of an indolent ulcer or corneal sequestrum. There is a rapid TBUT and decreased numbers of conjunctival goblet cells but aqueous tear production is normal.

- **Feline herpesvirus-1 (FHV-1) infection** FHV-1 invades the epithelia of the respiratory tract, conjunctiva, and to a lesser extent, the cornea. Primary infection is characterised by upper respiratory disease (coughing, sneezing, nasal discharge), lethargy, and pyrexia; ocular signs are bilateral conjunctivitis and corneal ulcers which can be bilateral. Herpetic ulcers tend to be dendritic or branching and are very painful. These lesions do not always breach the basement membrane of the corneal epithelium and as such will only stain with Rose Bengal and not with fluorescein dye (*Ch. 6, case 1, Fig. 6.1c*). Small corneal ulcers can rapidly coalesce to form large irregular areas of epithelial loss – this 'geographic' ulcer is the most common corneal lesion seen with FHV-1 infection. Following primary infection most cats became latent carriers and a proportion of carriers will develop conjunctivitis and/or corneal ulceration as adults because of recrudescence of the virus. In adult cats, conjunctivitis and/or ulcerative keratitis is mild and upper respiratory tract signs may not be present. Recurrent ocular signs are usually unilateral but can be bilateral; it is not uncommon for one eye to have repeat episodes whilst the other eye remains clinically normal.

- ***Chlamydophila felis (C felis)* infection** Chlamydiae are commensals of the ocular, respiratory, gastrointestinal and genital tracts, but cats infected with *C felis* rarely show systemic signs other than mild upper respiratory disease. The acute phase of the disease causes conjunctival hyperaemia, chemosis, serous ocular discharge and blepharospasm; nasal discharge and sneezing may also occur. Conjunctivitis is initially unilateral, becoming bilateral within several days. In contrast to FHV-1 infection, corneal involvement is not a feature of ocular chlamydophilosis. *C felis* can result in chronic conjunctivitis and an asymptomatic carrier state can exist.

- **Corneal sequestrum (corneal necrosis)** This is a common condition in the cat, particularly in the Persian, Himalayan and other brachycephalic breeds. Although a sequestrum is characterised by pathognomonic brown-to-black discolouration of the cornea (*Ch. 8, case 3*), the initial stage can be amber discolouration with concurrent ulceration. The amber discolouration can be overlooked, as it may only be evident with good magnification such as that provided by slit-lamp biomicroscopy. Pain is invariably present because of the corneal ulceration.

- **Trauma/foreign body** Blunt or penetrating trauma, and corneal or conjunctival foreign bodies can cause ocular pain and discharge. Clinical signs are usually acute and unilateral (*Ch. 12*). Cat fights are a common cause of corneal and conjunctival trauma.

- **Adnexal disorders**
  - **Eyelid agenesis or coloboma** This refers to a congenital absence of eyelid tissue, which may result in exposure of the ocular surface, trichiasis and a reduced ability to blink. Eyelid agenesis most commonly involves the lateral upper eyelid of cats and clinical signs occur at a young age. Cats with eyelid agenesis have conjunctivitis, keratitis and associated discomfort.
  - **Entropion** This refers to inversion or inward turning of part or all of the eyelid margin. Hair consequently contacts the ocular surface (trichiasis) and causes pain because of associated conjunctivitis, keratitis or corneal ulceration. Entropion is uncommon in the cat and is usually secondary to chronic blepharospasm or enophthalmos, the latter in geriatric cats because of orbital fat and muscle atrophy.
  - **Eyelash disorders** Ectopic cilia and distichiasis are rare in the cat (*Ch. 2, case 2; case 1, this chapter*).

3. Appropriate diagnostic tests

- Ocular reflexes
  - Pupillary light reflex – direct and consensual positive OU
  - Dazzle reflex – positive OU
  - Palpebral reflex – positive OU
- Menace response – positive OU
- Schirmer tear test – 17 mm/min OS, 10 mm/min OD. The marked difference (OS > OD) is suggestive of increased lacrimation in the left eye.
- Fluorescein dye
  - Staining – an irregular area of positive staining and under-running of dye in the lateral region of the cornea OS, negative OD (Fig. 5.2c, A). The under-running is consistent with non-adherent epithelium around the edge of the lesion.
  - Jones test (fluorescein dye passage test) – positive OU
  - Tear film break-up time – 3 s OS, 8 s OD. This is suggestive of reduced tear film stability in both eyes (OS > OD).

Examination of a painful eye can be facilitated by the topical application of a local anaesthetic drug. However topical anaesthetic drugs disrupt the tear film and are epitheliotoxic. They can temporarily decrease the tear film break-up time and can cause false-positive results with Rose Bengal and fluorescein stains. For these reasons, topical anaesthetic drugs should not be applied before these diagnostic tests.

- Tonometry – IOP 18 mmHg OU
- Polymerase chain reaction (PCR) assay – corneal and conjunctival swabs are negative for *C felis*, FHV-1 and feline calicivirus (FCV).

The diagnosis of FHV-1 can usually be based on clinical signs. Specific tests are available, e.g. conjunctival or corneal swab for PCR, but results often confuse rather than clarify the diagnosis. This is because PCR assays detect both vaccine and wild-type viral antigen and so their clinical use is questionable in a vaccinated cat (Maggs & Clarke, 2005).

Following topical anaesthesia, the posterior aspect of the TEL is examined for the presence of a foreign body and none is found. The remainder of the ophthalmic examination reveals no additional abnormalities and a general physical examination is unremarkable.

Diagnosis

Based on the information available, a diagnosis of an indolent corneal ulcer in the left eye is made. The ulcer appears to be secondary to a bilateral qualititative tear film deficiency. The subtle corneal opacity in the right eye represents a superficial scar from previous corneal disease.

Treatment

Indolent corneal ulcers can be treated medically or surgically. Surgical management is generally reserved for cats that do not respond to medical treatment. Debridement of the corneal ulcer is indicated to remove the non-adherent epithelium at the periphery and is usually performed under topical anaesthesia. Sedation or general anaesthesia may be required depending on the temperament of the cat and the skill of the clinician.

Topical anaesthesia is sufficient for this cat. A gentle dry debridement is performed in a circular motion with the tip of a sterile swab until all the non-adherent epithelium is removed. This creates a larger but still superficial ulcer (Fig. 5.2c, B). Following debridement a bandage contact lens is placed to improve comfort and facilitate healing (Fig. 5.2c, C). A single application of 0.5–1.0% topical atropine is administered to prevent the onset of reflex uveitis as a result of the debridement. Adjunctive medical management comprises a topical broad-spectrum antibiotic, a mucinomimetic agent, e.g. carbomer polymer gel, and systemic NSAID therapy.

Topical antibiotics have epitheliotoxic effects but the magnitude of the effect on epithelial healing depends on the specific drug. Gentamicin and ciprofloxacin are particularly epitheliotoxic and should be avoided in eyes with poor epithelial healing especially when alternative antibiotics, e.g. fusidic acid and chloramphenicol, are just as likely to be effective.

Atropine is a parasympatholytic agent with potent cycloplegic and mydriatic effects. It is indicated in the management of anterior uveitis, including reflex uveitis caused by ocular surface pain. However atropine also reduces tear production, which in turn can result in delayed corneal healing. Atropine should therefore be used with the minimal frequency required to maintain mydriasis.

Re-examination is performed after 48 hours. The corneal ulcer is significantly smaller (Fig. 5.2c, D), and heals completely by five days (Fig. 5.2c, E). Topical long-term mucinomimetic therapy is recommended in both eyes to address the underlying qualitative tear film deficiency.

Several techniques have been described to stimulate the healing of indolent ulcers in dogs including grid keratotomy, multiple punctate keratotomy and phenol cautery. These should not be performed in the cat because there is evidence to suggest that they predispose to the development of a corneal sequestrum. A superficial keratectomy, performed under general anaesthesia and with the aid of an operating microscope is, however, very successful in cats with indolent ulcers, as it is in dogs. In the cat, a superficial keratectomy results in a mean healing time of 14 days compared to 30 days with debridement of the cornea alone (La Croix et al., 2001).

Prognosis

The prognosis for the resolution of an indolent corneal ulcer secondary to a qualitative tear film disorder is only fair, because recurrence is not uncommon and surgical intervention may be necessary.

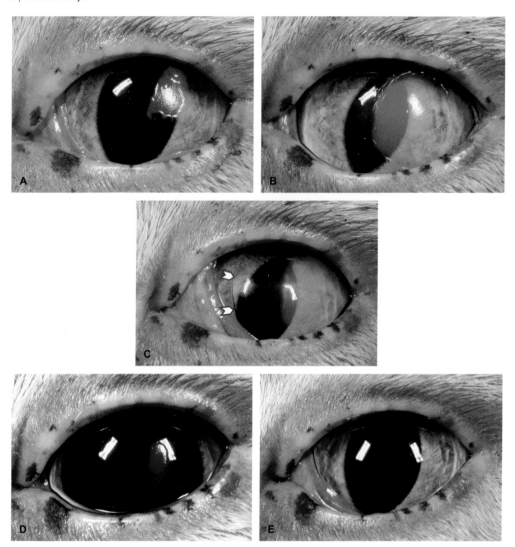

Fig. 5.2c (A) Corneal ulcer on presentation. (B) Increase in size of the ulcer following debridement. (C) Colourless bandage contact lens (arrows). (D) Decrease in size of the ulcer after 48 h (contact lens removed for examination). The pupil is dilated because of the topical application of atropine. (E) Ulcer healed after five days. Note the change in the Purkinje images throughout this series of photographs. The Purkinje images are initially disrupted when the ulcer is present but are more normal in (C) because of the 'masking' effect of the contact lens and in (E) when the ulcer has healed.

Discussion

The hallmark of an indolent or non-healing corneal ulcer is the presence of a rim of non-adherent epithelium surrounding a superficial ulcer. Indolent ulcers can be frustrating to manage and it is important to perform a thorough examination to try to identify a specific underlying cause. In the cat, causes include FHV-1 infection, trauma, and qualitative tear film disorders (mucin deficiency).

Conjunctival goblet cells are the primary source of mucin which forms the innermost layer of the tear film. Mucin also has a vital role in maintaining ocular surface health through corneal epithelial hydration, lubrication, and cleansing.

The diagnosis of a tear film disorder is usually made based on clinical signs but it can be difficult to differentiate qualitative from quantitative problems on this basis alone. A quantitative tear film disorder is a deficiency in the aqueous component of the tear film. By comparison, a qualitative tear film disorder refers to abnormal composition of the tear film. A quantitative tear film disorder is objectively diagnosed from the results of a Schirmer tear test, whereas a qualitative tear film disorder is objectively diagnosed from the TBUT, and less commonly, from the assessment of conjunctival goblet cell density (via a conjunctival biopsy and histopathology).

It is important to educate owners about the recurrent and possibly bilateral nature of indolent corneal ulcers and to choose treatment options that are appropriate for the species.

> A quantitative tear film disorder is a deficiency in the aqueous component of the tear film. By comparison, a qualitative tear film disorder refers to abnormal composition of the tear film.

References and further reading

Cullen CL, Njaa BL, Grahn BH (1999) Ulcerative keratitis associated with qualitative tear film abnormalities in cats. *Vet Ophthalmol*, **2**, 197–204.

La Croix NC, van der Woerdt A, Olivero DK (2001) Non-healing corneal ulcers in cats: 29 cases (1991–1999). *J Vet Med Assoc*, **218** (5) 733–750.

Maggs DJ & Clarke HE (2005) Relative sensitivity of polymerase chain reaction assays used for detection of feline herpesvirus-1 DNA in clinical samples and commercial vaccines. *Am J Vet Res*, **66** (9) 1550–1555.

See Appendix 2.

History

A three-year-old female neutered Jack Russell Terrier is presented with a 24-hour history of a painful right eye and a subdued demeanour. The dog has received routine vaccinations and anthelmintic treatment.

Questions

1. Describe the abnormalities and pertinent normal features in Figs. 5.3a and b.
2. What differential diagnoses should be considered for this presentation?
3. What tests could you perform to make the diagnosis?

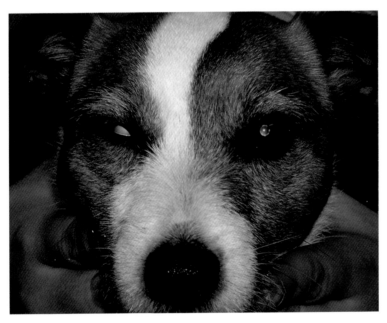

Fig. 5.3a

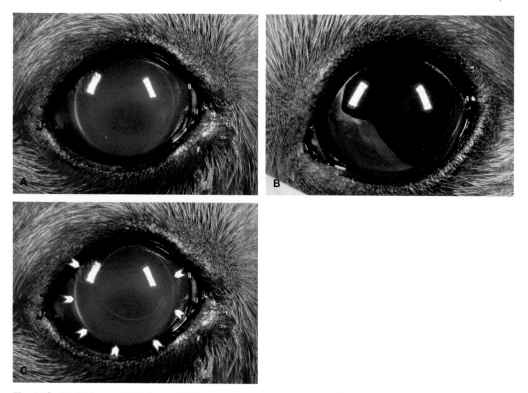

Fig. 5.3b (A) Right eye (B) Left eye (C) Right eye – the edge of the lens is delineated by arrows and the pupil is indicated by the circle.

Answers

1. What the figures show

Fig. 5.3a The left eye appears normal. Right eye – the palpebral fissure is narrow, and the pupil is dilated creating a relative anisocoria (OD > OS).

Fig. 5.3b Right eye (A) – there is dried ocular discharge adjacent to the medial canthus and diffuse corneal oedema. A spherical refractile structure (lens) is visible in the anterior chamber (see annotated image, C). The Purkinje images are normal. Left eye (B) – there are iris-to-iris persistent pupillary membrane remnants and light grey, fine wispy strands within the pupil and overlying the iris. The Purkinje images are normal. The reflection of the photographer's finger is evident in the medial cornea.

2. Differential diagnoses

Given the history and appearance of the right eye, the following conditions should be considered:

- **Anterior lens luxation** This most commonly occurs as a primary heritable condition in terriers and other predisposed breeds, e.g. Border Collie, Shar Pei, German Shepherd Dog and some spaniel breeds. Primary lens luxation is a bilateral condition, but both eyes are not necessarily involved simultaneously. The most common clinical presentation for an anterior lens luxation is acute pain in one eye in a three- to six-year-old dog. The pain is the result of entrapment of the lens in the anterior chamber which in turn causes an acute elevation in IOP. Other clinical signs include epiphora, blepharospasm, corneal oedema, episcleral congestion and a change in anterior chamber depth. The lens may or may not be visible in the anterior chamber depending on the degree of corneal oedema. Very occasionally, the lens loses its zonular attachments but remains behind the pupil – from this position it can push the iris forward and create a shallow anterior chamber. Examination of the contralateral eye often reveals signs of lens subluxation (partial detachment of lens zonules), e.g. strands of degenerate vitreous material in the anterior chamber, phacodonesis, iridodonesis, and an aphakic crescent. Secondary causes of lens luxation in the dog are also common. These include trauma (usually associated with profound ocular injury), age-related degeneration of the lens zonules, hypermature cataract, buphthalmos (causes stretching and tearing of the lens zonules), and physical displacement of the lens by an intraocular neoplasm. Congenital lens luxation is reported in the dog but is rare.

- **Glaucoma** This term describes a group of related ocular diseases with the common factors of reduced aqueous humor drainage from the eye and optic nerve damage. In dogs this is usually associated with an elevation in IOP. Causes of glaucoma can be classified as primary, secondary or congenital. Primary glaucoma is thought to arise from an inherent abnormality with the aqueous humour outflow system, and includes pectinate ligament dysplasia (goniodysgenesis). Glaucoma can be secondary to chronic or severe ocular disease e.g uveitis, lens luxation, intraocular neoplasia. Congenital glaucoma is rare in the dog. In addition to an elevation in IOP, classic signs of acute glaucoma include discomfort, episcleral congestion, mydriasis, corneal oedema, reduced vision, optic disc abnormalities (swelling, cupping, degeneration) and retinal changes (*Ch. 6, case 2*). Signs of chronic glaucoma include buphthalmos, episcleral congestion, corneal oedema, Haab's striae, keratitis, mydriasis, lens subluxation, optic nerve and retinal degeneration, blindness and discomfort.

- **Uveitis** Inflammation of the uveal tract can involve the entire uvea (panuveitis) but is usually confined to either the anterior (iris and ciliary body) or posterior (choroid) regions of the uvea. Inflammation of the uveal tract reflects the fact that it is the primary vascular source of the eye. The uvea forms a blood-aqueous barrier which consists of the non-pigmented epithelium of the ciliary body and the endothelium of the blood vessels of the iris. Anterior uveitis occurs when the integrity of the blood-aqueous barrier is compromised. The aetiopathogenesis of uveitis is complex. Examples of ocular causes of uveitis include corneal ulcer (reflex uveitis), cataract (lens-induced uveitis), primary intraocular neoplasia and trauma. Systemic causes include immune-mediated disease (e.g. Vogt-Koyanagi-Harada-like or uveodermatologic syndrome), metastatic neoplasia and infectious disease: viral (e.g. infectious canine hepatitis), bacterial (e.g. *Leptospira* sp), fungal (e.g. *Blastomyces dermatitidis*), rickettsial (e.g. *Ehrlichia canis*), protozoal (*Toxoplasma gondii*), and parasitic (*Dirofilaria immitis*). The clinical features of uveitis depend on the area of the uvea involved, the severity of the inflammation and whether the process is acute or chronic. Acute anterior uveitis is characterised by discomfort (blepharospasm, increased lacrimation and photophobia), conjunctival and episcleral congestion, ciliary flush, miosis, hypotony, protein and cells in the aqueous humour (aqueous flare, hypopyon, hyphaema, fibrin) and corneal oedema (*Ch. 7, cases 2 and 3*).

- **Ocular surface pain** See cases 1 and 2, this chapter; Ch. 2, Ch. 8 (case 3), and Ch. 12.

> Ocular discomfort, redness and corneal oedema are common to both uveitis and glaucoma but the treatment and prognosis is quite different for each.

3. Appropriate diagnostic tests
- Ocular reflexes
  - Pupillary light reflex – positive direct and negative consensual OS (from left to right eye); negative direct and positive consensual OD (right to left eye)

○ Dazzle reflex – positive OU
○ Palpebral reflex – positive OU
- Vision testing
  ○ Menace response – positive OS, negative OD
  ○ Visual placing and tracking reflexes – positive OS, negative OD

In this dog, the findings suggest that there is a visual deficit in the right eye but that retinal and optic nerve function is still intact. The lack of pupil constriction in the right eye may be attributed to the presence of the lens in the anterior chamber.

- Examination with a focal light source – slit-lamp biomicroscopy reveals phacodonesis and iridodonesis in the left eye.
- Ophthalmoscopy – normal fundus OS. Corneal oedema and the presence of the lens in the anterior chamber prevent fundic examination OD.
- Schirmer tear test – 18 mm/min OS, 23 mm/min OD
- Fluorescein dye – negative staining OS, mild diffuse retention OD which is evident only after several minutes.
- Tonometry – IOP 20 mmHg OS, 35 mmHg OD
- Gonioscopy – normal filtration angle OS. This is not performed in the right eye because the corneal oedema would prevent observation of the filtration angle.

A functional corneal endothelium is vital for maintenance of corneal transparency. Corneal oedema develops secondary to an anterior lens luxation for two main reasons. Firstly, the physical contact between the lens and the corneal endothelium causes focal oedema (typically subaxial). Secondly, generalised corneal oedema results from the increased intraocular pressure and anterior uveitis caused by the lens movement. Corneal oedema can cause subtle focal or diffuse fluorescein retention, indicative of the reduced integrity of the epithelial barrier rather than actual corneal ulceration.

The remainder of the ophthalmic examination reveals no additional abnormalities and a general physical examination is unremarkable.

Diagnosis

Based on the information available, a diagnosis of primary lens luxation is made – anterior lens luxation and secondary glaucoma in the right eye and lens subluxation in the left eye.

Treatment

Prompt surgical treatment is important if the eye with an anterior lens luxation is determined to be visual or is considered to have the potential for vision. The potential for vision is best determined following consideration of the duration of clinical signs, the severity of secondary glaucoma and the presence or absence of a dazzle reflex and consensual pupillary light reflex. Standard vision assessment tests are frequently unhelpful because of pain, corneal oedema and elevated IOP (causing neuropraxia). An intracapsular lens extraction (ICLE), with or without artificial lens implantation, is the treatment of choice. If the eye is determined to be irreversibly blind, surgical options are restricted to enucleation or the placement of an intrascleral prosthesis. There is considerable diversity of opinion amongst veterinary ophthalmologists about the best management strategy for a subluxated lens. Primary lens luxation is a bilateral condition and an unstable lens in the fellow eye will eventually luxate completely either anteriorly or posteriorly. The interval between the first and

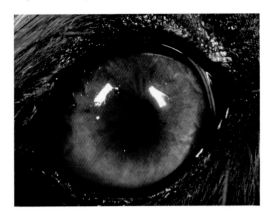

Fig. 5.3c Miosis following topical therapy with travoprost, a prostaglandin analogue.

second eye being affected is often impossible to predict. Some ophthalmologists advocate long-term topical miotic therapy to reduce the risk of the lens moving forwards into the anterior chamber. Lens instability is also associated with mild elevations in IOP and potent miotics (such as the prostaglandin analogues latanoprost or travoprost) will also reduce IOP (Fig. 5.3c). An alternative approach is prophylactic lentectomy by phacoemulsification or ICLE, with or without artificial lens implantation. A good success rate for early surgical intervention has been documented by some authors but early surgery carries the risk of premature blindness from complications such as retinal detachment and intraocular haemorrhage.

This dog is managed by an ICLE in the right eye and prophylactic phacoemulsification (facilitated by placement of a capsule tension ring) in the left eye. This results in aphakic vision in both eyes. Postoperative medication consists of topical steroid and antibiotic therapy, and systemic NSAID and antibiotic therapy. Long-term monitoring is also recommended.

Prognosis

The prognosis for vision and for the eye itself is guarded following surgical removal of an anterior luxated lens. The most common complications include the development of glaucoma and retinal detachment. Irreversible blindness and pain frequently necessitate enucleation or placement of an intrascleral prosthesis. The prognosis for vision after ICLE is considered poor if glaucoma is already present at the time of surgery, an inevitable finding in the majority of cases of anterior lens luxation. The decision regarding management of subluxated lenses is challenging. A retrospective study in dogs showed that the prognosis for vision was significantly greater if the lens was removed by phacoemulsification rather than ICLE. In that study, 75% of eyes were visual 2.75 years following phacolentectomy, compared to 40% of eyes following ICLE at the same time period (Manning et al., 2008; Fig. 5.3d). The long-term efficacy of miotic therapy is currently unknown so it is impossible to make further comparisons.

Discussion

Primary lens luxation is a complex condition related to an inherited dysplasia and weakening of the lens zonules. Even with prompt and appropriate management, the prognosis for vision is guarded. The diagnosis can be challenging because the clinical presentation is not dissimilar to other painful ocular conditions such as acute glaucoma and anterior uveitis. Accurate diagnosis is imperative and is aided by knowledge of breed predisposition. Terriers are the most common breeds affected and lens luxation should be considered in all terriers which present with an acutely painful eye. Terrier breeds are also predisposed to primary glaucoma and the two conditions can co-exist.

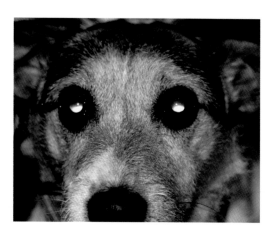

Fig. 5.3d An eight-year-old Jack Russell Terrier with bilateral aphakic vision and normotensive eyes three years after surgery – ICLE for an anterior lens luxation in the right eye and prophylactic phacoemulsification for lens subluxation in the left eye.

Furthermore, chronic glaucoma often results in buphthalmos (*Ch. 1, case 1*) – globe enlargement causes stretching of the lens zonules and secondary lens subluxation. Identification of the primary problem can therefore be difficult in a terrier breed with concurrent lens subluxation and an elevated IOP. Diagnosis of lens luxation is facilitated by tonometry, gonioscopy and slit-lamp biomicroscopy. It is particularly important to perform a careful examination of the contralateral eye to look for signs of early subluxation. The pupil should first be dilated with a short-acting mydriatic, e.g. tropicamide, because it is easier to identify early signs of lens instability such as vitreal strands and an aphakic crescent through a dilated pupil. Dilating the pupil is not without risk as mydriasis can increase IOP or facilitate movement of the lens into the anterior chamber.

Primary lens luxation has been determined to be heritable in some breeds and a DNA test for terriers has recently become available. Affected dogs should not be used for breeding.

References and further reading

Manning S, Renwick P, Heinrich C, Cripps P. (2009) Lens instability in the dog: a retrospective study of surgical results in 102 cases (155 eyes) (1994–2004). Proc Eur Coll Vet Ophthalmol, Versailles 2008, *Vet Ophthalmol*, **12** (1), 61–70.

See Appendix 2.

CHAPTER 6

The Red Eye

Introduction

An eye may appear red for a variety of reasons; inflammation or congestion of the conjunctiva, sclera and uvea is common but the cornea and anterior chamber may also be involved. A red appearance usually suggests an ocular abnormality, but it can be a normal variation, e.g. a red reflection from a subalbinotic fundus. Owners often assume ocular redness means pain, but this is not always true.

Small Animal Ophthalmology: What's Your Diagnosis? First Edition. Heidi Featherstone, Elaine Holt.
© 2011 by Heidi Featherstone and Elaine Holt. Published 2011 by Blackwell Publishing Ltd.

History

A 9-month-old female neutered domestic shorthaired cat is presented with a four-day history of redness and discharge in the right eye. The cat has been sneezing occasionally but is reported to be otherwise well. She has received anthelmintic treatment but has never been vaccinated. She lives with another young adult cat who has been routinely vaccinated; both are indoor/outdoor cats.

Questions

1. Describe the abnormalities and pertinent normal features in Fig. 6.1a.
2. What differential diagnoses should be considered for this presentation?
3. What tests could you perform to make the diagnosis?

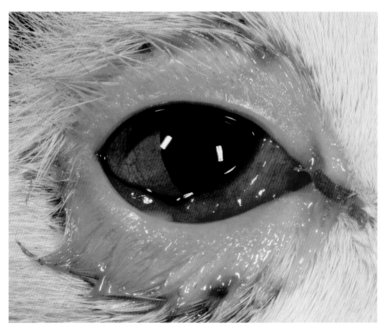

Fig. 6.1a

Answers

1. What the figure shows?

Fig. 6.1a Right eye – there is hyperaemia and chemosis of the palpebral and TEL conjunctiva and a marked seromucoid ocular discharge. The Purkinje images are normal.

2. Differential diagnoses

Given the appearance of the right eye, the clinical diagnosis is conjunctivitis. The following causes should be considered:

- **Feline herpesvirus-1 infection** FHV-1 invades the epithelia of the respiratory tract, conjunctiva and, to a lesser effect, the cornea. Primary infection is characterised by upper respiratory disease (coughing, sneezing, nasal discharge), lethargy, and pyrexia; ocular signs are bilateral conjunctivitis and corneal ulcers which can be bilateral. Herpetic ulcers tend to be dendritic or branching and can be painful. These lesions do not always breach the basement membrane of the corneal epithelium and as such will only stain with rose Bengal and not with fluorescein dye (*Figs. 6.1b and c*). Small corneal ulcers can rapidly coalesce to form a large irregular area of epithelial loss – this 'geographic' ulcer is the most common corneal lesion seen with FHV-1 infection. Following primary infection most cats become latent carriers and a proportion of carriers will develop conjunctivitis and/or corneal ulceration as adults because of recrudescence of the virus. In adult cats, conjunctivitis and/or ulcerative keratitis is mild and upper respiratory tract signs may not be present. Recurrent ocular signs are usually unilateral in adult cats but can be bilateral; it is not uncommon for one eye to have repeat episodes while the other eye remains clinically normal.
- *Chlamydophila felis* **infection** Chlamydiae are commensals of the ocular, respiratory, gastrointestinal and genital tracts, but cats infected with *C felis* rarely show systemic signs other than mild upper respiratory disease. The acute phase of the disease causes conjunctival hyperaemia, chemosis, serous ocular discharge and blepharospasm; nasal discharge and sneezing may also occur. Conjunctivitis is initially unilateral, becoming bilateral within several days. In contrast to FHV-1 infection, corneal involvement is not a feature of ocular chlamydophilosis. *C felis* can result in chronic conjunctivitis and an asymptomatic carrier state can exist.
- **Feline calicivirus infection** FCV is primarily a respiratory pathogen but can cause conjunctivitis, oral ulceration and polyarthritis. In contrast to *C felis* and FHV-1, FCV has a low pathogenicity for the conjunctiva. Most cats recover spontaneously from FCV infection, although some cats remain chronically infected and shed virus continuously.
- **Eosinophilic conjunctivitis** This may occur alone or in conjunction with eosinophilic keratitis; it can be unilateral or bilateral. The underlying cause is unknown. Diagnosis is confirmed by the identification of eosinophils on conjunctival cytology.
- **Lipogranulomatous conjunctivitis** This condition is specific to the cat and is characterised by non-ulcerated, single or multiple white nodules in the palpebral conjunctiva adjacent to the eyelid margin. The condition is often bilateral and can involve both the upper and, less frequently, lower eyelids. Diagnosis is based on the clinical appearance and histopathology to confirm the presence of lipogranulomatous inflammation associated with intact or ruptured meibomian glands.
- **Mycoplasmosis** The role of a *Mycoplasma* sp as a cause of conjunctivitis in cats is unclear; the organism can be isolated from healthy cats as well as from cats with conjunctivitis (Low *et al.*, 2007). Experimental infection has only resulted in conjunctivitis in kittens and not in adult cats, which suggests an altered or immature immune system may be a factor in establishment of infection. Diagnosis is by conjunctival cytology, culture and/or PCR, but testing is not indicated in clinical cases of conjunctivitis.
- **Bordetellosis** *Bordetella bronchiseptica* is a respiratory pathogen in the cat which can cause upper respiratory signs and conjunctivitis. In contrast to the dog, clinical disease in the cat is rare but

cats from multicat housing conditions such as catteries and shelters are predisposed. Diagnosis is by conjunctival culture but testing is rarely indicated in clinical cases of conjunctivitis.
- **Parasitic conjunctivitis** A rare cause of conjunctivitis in the cat, e.g. nematode *Thelazia californiensis* and larvae of *Cuterebra* sp.

3. Appropriate diagnostic tests
- Ocular reflexes
  - ○ Pupillary light reflex – direct and consensual positive OU
  - ○ Dazzle reflex – positive OU
- Menace response – positive OU
- Examination with a focal light source – slit-lamp biomicroscopy reveals no corneal abnormalities before or after the application of fluorescein and rose Bengal dye (see below).
- Schirmer tear test – 10 mm/min OS. Tear production is not measured OD because of the excessive lacrimation.
- Fluorescein dye – negative staining OU (Fig. 6.1b)
- Rose Bengal dye – negative staining OU (Fig. 6.1c)

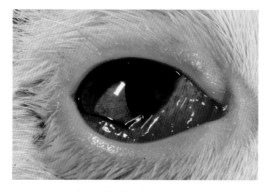

Fig. 6.1b Right eye following application of fluorescein dye. There is no dye retention.

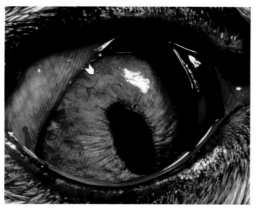

Fig. 6.1c Right eye of a different adult cat following the application of fluorescein and Rose Bengal dyes. Retention of Rose Bengal dye in a branching pattern (arrow) indicates dendritic corneal ulceration which is pathognomonic for FHV-1 infection.

Rose Bengal is an ocular surface stain the uptake of which is normally blocked by mucin in the tear film. Stain retention therefore represents poor stability of the tear film and suboptimal protection of the epithelium. Rose Bengal staining is indicated for the diagnosis of corneal erosions caused by FHV-1 which are often negative following fluorescein staining (Fig. 6.1c). Rose Bengal and fluorescein can be administered at the same time as the stain properties are not affected by mixing.

- Tonometry – IOP 18 mmHg OU
- Cytology (conjunctiva) – this reveals epithelial cells and degenerate neutrophils, and a conspicuous absence of eosinophils and *C felis* inclusion bodies.
- Culture and sensitivity (conjunctiva) – this reveals a moderate growth of *Staphylococcus* sp sensitive to most routine antibiotics.
- PCR – a conjunctival swab is positive for *C felis* but negative for FHV-1 and FCV.

The remainder of the ophthalmic examination reveals no additional abnormalities and a general physical examination is unremarkable.

Diagnosis

Based on the information available, a diagnosis of conjunctivitis in the right eye secondary to *Chlamydophila felis* infection is made.

Treatment

Systemic treatment of *C felis* is indicated even if the disease is clinically restricted to the eye because chlamydiae are commensals of the ocular, respiratory, gastrointestinal and genital tracts. The drug of choice is systemic doxycyline 5 mg/kg twice daily for three weeks. Topical 1% fusidic acid or 1% chlortetracycline have been shown to be less effective than systemic doxycyline in the treatment of feline chlamydiosis (Sparkes *et al.,* 1999). Topical antibiotic therapy can, however, be beneficial for the treatment of any secondary bacterial infections that may be present concurrently. Systemic doxycyline should bring a rapid improvement of the clinical signs and should eradicate the organism. To minimise the risk of doxycycline-induced oesophagitis and stricture formation, a suspension should be used or, if unavailable, tablet administration followed by a water bolus given by syringe. All cats in a multicat household should be treated at the same time to prevent re-infection.

Studies have evaluated systemic antibiotics for the treatment of feline chlamydiosis. Oral clavulanic acid-potentiated amoxicillin and azithromycin are both as effective as oral doxycycline in improving clinical signs and reducing isolation of the organism, but do not eliminate the organism allowing recurrence of clinical signs (Sturgess *et al.,* 2001; Owen *et al.,* 2003).

Prognosis

The prognosis for resolution of the conjunctivitis without recurrence as a result of *C felis* infection is excellent with appropriate treatment.

Discussion

Feline conjunctivitis is a very common ocular disease and, in contrast to condition in the dog, is usually infectious in origin. Specific identification of the two most common infectious causes, FHV-1 and *C felis*, is often challenging and co-infection is possible though uncommon. An important difference between the two agents is the ability of FHV-1 to infect the corneal epithelium. Because of this, a cat with unilateral conjunctivitis and concurrent corneal ulceration is more likely to have FHV-1 than *C felis*. PCR assays are helpful in the diagnosis of feline chlamydophilosis but are of questionable value for FHV-1 in vaccinated cats or cats with chronic disease (Maggs & Clarke, 2005). Conjunctival cytology is an unreliable method of diagnosis for *C felis* because the characteristic inclusion bodies are only present from day three after infection and decrease in number over the following two weeks. Inclusion bodies can also be confused with 'blue bodies' which represent epithelial cell inclusion bodies caused by topical medications such as neomycin. Routine vaccination with a live *C felis* vaccine is effective at reducing the severity of ocular disease but has no effect on shedding of the organism or its ability to infect and persist in non-ocular sites e.g. genital tract. The vaccine can also cause atypical reactions and is usually reserved for use in control programmes in catteries with a high prevalence of systemic chlamydophilosis.

References and further reading

Low HC, Powell CC, Veir JK, Hawley JR, Lappin MR (2007) Prevalence of feline herpesvirus 1, *Chlamydophila felis*, and *Mycoplasma* spp DNA in conjunctival cells collected from cats with and without conjunctivitis. *Am J Vet Res*, **68** (6), 643–648.

Maggs DJ & Clarke HE (2005) Relative sensitivity of polymerase chain reaction assays used for detection of feline herpesvirus type 1 DNA in clinical samples and commercial vaccines. *Am J Vet Res*, **66** (9), 1550–1555.

Owen WMA, Sturgess CP, Harbour DA, Egan K, Gruffydd-Jones TJ (2003) Efficacy of azithromycin for the treatment of feline chlamydophilosis. *J Feline Med Surg*, **5** (6), 305–311.

Sparkes AH, Caney SMA, Sturgess CP, Gruffydd-Jones TJ (1999) The clinical efficacy of topical and systemic therapy for the treatment of feline ocular chlamydiosis. *J Feline Med Surg*, **1** (1), 31–35.

See Appendix 2.

History

A 6-year-old male neutered Basset hound is presented with a 48-hour history of acute redness and haziness in the left eye. The dog has been sleeping more than usual and resents the owner touching the affected eye. He has received routine vaccinations and anthelmintic treatment and is reportedly otherwise well.

Questions

1. Describe the abnormalities and pertinent normal features in Fig. 6.2a.
2. What differential diagnosis should be considered for this presentation?
3. What tests could you perform to make the diagnosis?

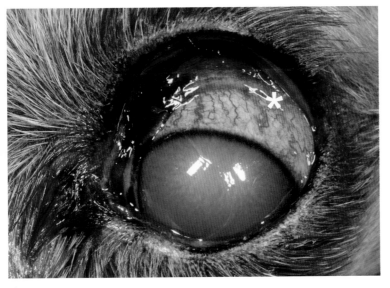

Fig. 6.2a

Answers

1. What the figure shows

Fig. 6.2a Left eye (the upper eyelid is manually elevated) – there is a serous ocular discharge at the medial canthus, generalised corneal opacification, and marked conjunctival and episcleral congestion. The Purkinje images are disrupted because of a strand of mucus on the cornea. The free margin of the TEL is pigmented and continues circumferentially around the globe posterior to the limbus (asterix) – this represents an encircling TEL which is common in some dog breeds (e.g. American Cocker Spaniel) and is considered to be clinically insignificant.

2. Differential diagnoses

Given the appearance of the left eye, the following conditions should be considered:

- **Glaucoma** This term describes a group of related ocular diseases with the common factors of reduced aqueous humour drainage from the eye and optic nerve damage. In dogs this is usually associated with an elevation in IOP. Causes of glaucoma can be classified as primary, secondary or congenital. Primary glaucoma is thought to arise from an inherent abnormality with the aqueous humour outflow system, and includes pectinate ligament dysplasia (goniodysgenesis). Glaucoma can be secondary to chronic or severe ocular disease, e.g. uveitis, lens luxation, intraocular neoplasia. Congenital glaucoma is rare in the dog. In addition to an elevation in IOP, classic signs of acute glaucoma include discomfort, episcleral congestion, mydriasis, corneal oedema, reduced vision, optic disc abnormalities (swelling, cupping, degeneration) and retinal changes. Signs of chronic glaucoma include buphthalmos, episcleral congestion, corneal oedema, Haab's striae, keratitis, mydriasis, lens subluxation, optic nerve and retinal degeneration, blindness and discomfort.

- **Anterior uveitis** Inflammation of the uveal tract can involve the entire uvea (panuveitis) but is usually confined to either the anterior (iris and ciliary body) or posterior (choroid) regions. Inflammation of the uveal tract reflects the fact that it is the primary vascular source of the eye. The uvea forms a blood-aqueous barrier which consists of the non-pigmented epithelium of the ciliary body and the endothelium of the blood vessels of the iris. Anterior uveitis occurs when the integrity of the blood-aqueous barrier is compromised. The aetiopathogenesis of uveitis is complex. Systemic causes include immune-mediated disease (e.g. Vogt-Koyanagi-Harada-like or uveodermatologic syndrome), metastatic neoplasia and infectious disease: viral (e.g. infectious canine hepatitis), bacterial (e.g. *Leptospira* sp), fungal (e.g. *Blastomyces dermatitidis*), rickettsial (e.g. *Ehrlichia canis*), protozoal (*Toxoplasma gondii*), or parasitic (*Dirofilaria immitis*). The clinical features of uveitis depend on the area of the uvea involved, the severity of the inflammation and whether the process is acute or chronic. Acute anterior uveitis is characterised by discomfort (blepharospasm, increased lacrimation and photophobia), conjunctival and episcleral congestion, ciliary flush, miosis, hypotony, protein and cells in the aqueous humour (aqueous flare, hypopyon, hyphaema, fibrin) and corneal oedema (*Ch. 7, cases 2 and 3*).

Ocular discomfort, redness and corneal oedema are common to both uveitis and glaucoma but the treatment and prognosis is quite different for each.

3. Appropriate diagnostic tests

- Ocular reflexes
  - Pupillary light reflex – negative direct and consensual OS (left to right eye); positive direct and negative consensual OD (right to left eye)
  - Dazzle reflex – negative OS, positive OD

- Vision assessment
  - Menace response – negative OS, positive OD
  - Visual placing and tracking reflexes negative OS, positive OD
  - Obstacle course – this dog can navigate around large objects in both photopic and scotopic conditions when the left eye is covered but is reluctant to move when the right eye is covered.

In this dog, these results are consistent with a blind left eye, and no sign of retinal and optic nerve function. The pupil in the left eye cannot constrict (see below).

- Examination with a focal light source – slit-lamp biomicroscopy reveals increased corneal thickness secondary to the oedema.

Pupil size provides helpful information about the presence and type of intraocular disease. The pupil is more likely to be dilated in an eye with glaucoma but miotic with anterior uveitis. Even in the presence of corneal opacity, pupil size can be assessed by illuminating the anterior segment from oblique angles in an attempt to detect a tapetal reflection.

- Ophthalmoscopy – fundic examination is not possible because of the generalised corneal oedema OS; the fundus OD is unremarkable.
- Schirmer tear test – 23 mm/min OS, 17 mm/min OD
- Fluorescein dye – negative staining OU
- Tonometry – IOP 53 mmHg OS, 20 mmHg OD. The elevated IOP in the right eye is the reason for the absent PLR because of damage to the optic nerve and retina, as well as hypoxia of the iris.
- Gonioscopy – severe pectinate ligament dysplasia manifested by flow holes (arrow) within extensive sheets of tissue is observed OD (Fig. 6.2b, A and Diagram 6.2). In the normal dog, distinct individual pectinate ligaments are seen (Fig. 6.2b, B and Diagram 6.2). Gonioscopy is not performed OS because of the corneal opacification.

Topical 2.5% phenylephrine is applied to the left eye – the conjunctival vessels blanch within several seconds, leaving the congested episcleral veins visible (Fig. 6.2c). The remainder of the ophthalmic examination reveals no additional abnormalities and a general physical examination is unremarkable.

When evaluating a 'red eye', it can be helpful to establish whether the blood vessel congestion/hyperaemia is superficial (conjunctival) or both superficial and deep (episcleral and scleral). Episcleral and scleral congestion/hyperaemia is usually associated with intraocular disease such as uveitis and glaucoma whereas conjunctival involvement alone suggests ocular surface disease. The conjunctival blood vessels are bright red, branching, tortuous, and mobile but vasoconstrict within several seconds of the topical application of a sympathomimetic such as phenylephrine or epinephrine. Deeper episcleral blood vessels are dark red, straight, and perpendicular to the limbus; single vessels can easily be distinguished and do not vasoconstrict rapidly following the application of topical phenylephrine or epinephrine.

Diagnosis

Based on the information available, a diagnosis of acute primary glaucoma is made in the left eye and goniodysgenesis in the right eye.

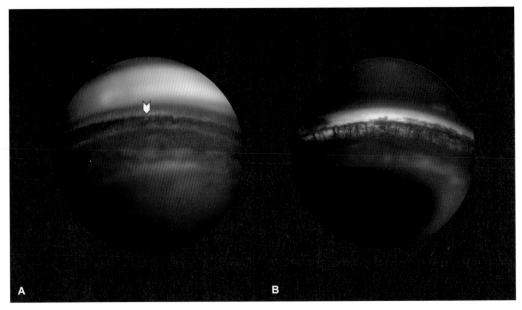

Fig. 6.2b (A) Severe pectinate ligament dysplasia (left eye). There are several flow holes (arrow) within abnormal tissue spanning the filtration angle. (B) Normal filtration angle in an adult Labrador Retriever for comparison.

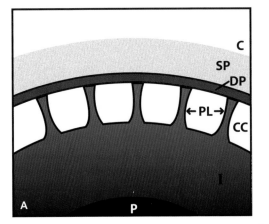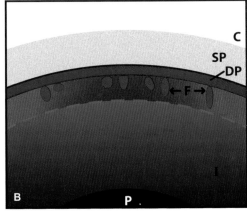

Diagram 6.2 (A) Gonioscopic view of normal canine filtration angle. (B) Gonioscopic view of canine filtration angle with goniodysgenesis (pectinate ligament dysplasia); C, cornea; SP, superficial pigmented zone; DP, deep pigmented zone; PL, pectinate ligaments; CC, ciliary cleft; I, iris; P, pupil; F, flow hole. Illustration by S Scurrell.

Treatment

The primary aim of the treatment of acute glaucoma is the rapid reduction of IOP to within a safe target range (<20 mmHg). Lowering IOP can be achieved by medical or surgical treatment, or a combination of both. The choice of treatment depends on the potential for vision, owner compliance, financial considerations and the temperament of the dog. There is no single effective medical treatment regimen for glaucoma. A treatment protocol for acute primary glaucoma includes a topical prostaglandin, e.g. latanoprost (an analogue of PGF2α) or travoprost. When applied topi-

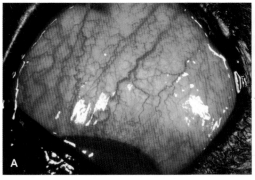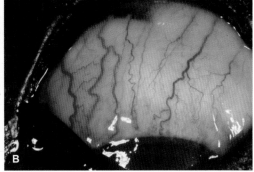

Fig. 6.2c (A) Marked conjunctival and episcleral congestion in the right eye. (B) Same eye several seconds after the topical application of 2.5% phenylephrine – the superficial vessels in the conjunctiva have blanched (because of vasoconstriction), making the deeper episcleral vessels more visible.

cally in very low concentrations these drugs are thought to lower the IOP in the dog by reducing aqueous humour production and/or increasing unconventional uveoscleral outflow (Miller *et al.*, 2010). Analgesia and anti-inflammatory therapy is also essential.

This dog initially receives 0.004% travoprost in the right eye and systemic NSAID therapy. The IOP is successfully lowered to 15 mmHg within one hour of treatment but the menace response and dazzle reflex remain absent. Treatment is continued with travoprost q12 hours, 2% brinzolamide q8 hours, and systemic NSAID therapy. Regular monitoring is performed to ensure that the IOP remains <20 mmHg. The eye does not regain vision and the IOP is 60 mmHg three weeks later. Enucleation is performed as the eye is considered to be irreversibly blind and painful. The diagnosis of goniodysgenesis and irreversible damage to the optic nerve (optic nerve 'cupping') is confirmed on histopathology (Fig. 6.2d).

Prophylactic treatment with a topical β-blocker is recommended for the contralateral eye. One study has shown that prophylactic treatment can delay the onset of the disease in the fellow eye by almost two years (Miller *et al.*, 2000). The right eye is treated with 0.5% timolol q12 hours and is re-examined every three months.

Many topical medications are available for the treatment of glaucoma in the dog. In addition to the aforementioned prostaglandins (e.g. latanoprost, travoprost) and β-blockers (e.g. timolol), there are miotics (e.g. pilocarpine), α-agonists (apraclonidine) and carbonic anhydrase inhibitors (e.g. brinzolamide, dorzolamide). The reader is directed to more detailed sources of information on the efficacy of these drugs. However, in general terms, prostaglandins are appropriate for acute primary glaucoma in the dog as they can successfully and rapidly lower a high IOP to a safe level. Prostaglandins induce a marked miosis in the dog and are therefore contraindicated in eyes with acute uveitis and anterior lens luxation. In comparison, carbonic anhydrase inhibitors take several days to reach their maximum effect and lower the IOP only slightly – as such they are more appropriate in an eye with a mildly elevated IOP. Systemic medications are now used infrequently and include hyperosmotic agents e.g. mannitol. These drugs are now only commonly used prior to glaucoma surgery. The role of neuroprotective drugs is currently under investigation. The term 'neuroprotection' refers to the protection of remaining retinal ganglion cells which have not been damaged by the elevated IOP.

Surgical treatment is available for primary glaucoma. Some procedures involve the creation of an alternative drainage pathway for aqueous humour, e.g. anterior chamber shunts, while others focus on decreasing the formation of aqueous humour, e.g. destruction of part of the ciliary body by laser or cryotherapy. Currently, the most frequently employed surgical techniques in veterinary medicine include gonioimplants (i.e. anterior chamber shunts), laser photocoagulation and cyclocryotherapy. The ideal surgical candidate still has vision and is in the early stages of glaucoma, i.e. the eye has a normal-appearing optic nerve head and no signs of uveitis or lens subluxation. Surgery to reduce IOP is not elected in this dog because the right eye remains blind even when it becomes normotensive.

Optic nerve axons are acutely sensitive to elevations in IOP. The normal IOP range in the dog is 15–25 mmHg. Even at 25 mmHg, 10% of the axons suffer adverse effects, and this increases to 100% at 50 mmHg. Once the optic nerve is damaged, the remaining axons are more sensitive to further IOP elevations. The 'safe' IOP for the dog is unknown, but general guidelines are 30 mmHg to maintain comfort, and <20 mmHg to maintain vision.

Prognosis

The long-term prognosis for a visual, comfortable eye is poor. The majority of dogs with primary glaucoma become blind and the eye continues to be painful despite appropriate medical therapy.

Vision after combined surgery with a gonioimplant and cyclophotocoagulation or cryotherapy has been reported to be present in 41–60% of dogs after one year (Bentley *et al.*, 1999; Sapienza & van der Woerdt, 2005). There is currently no published reports on the prognosis for vision with medical management alone compared with a combination of medical and surgical management.

Discussion

The canine glaucomas are a large and complex group of important ocular diseases. With primary glaucoma, the risk of permanent blindness is high because the disease is often not recognised until there is an acute onset of elevated IOP. Blindness results from damage to the retina and the optic nerve – the nerve may recover to a degree if prompt appropriate treatment is given, but irreversible optic nerve atrophy is common. The diagnosis of glaucoma is often delayed because of a low index of suspicion on the part of the owner and the veterinary surgeon. Primary glaucoma is most common in middle-aged pure-breed dogs e.g. Cocker Spaniel (American and English),

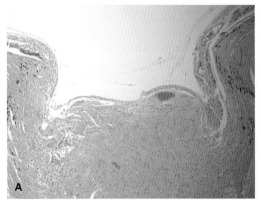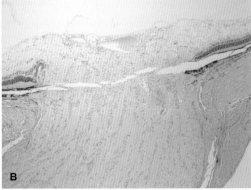

Fig. 6.2d (A) Atrophy of the optic nerve head characterised by marked 'cupping'. (B) Normal canine optic nerve head. (H & E, × 40). Reproduced with permission from EJ Scurrell.

Springer Spaniel (Welsh and English), Basset Hound, Chow Chow, Shar Pei, Wire-haired Fox Terrier, Norwegian Elkhound, Siberian Husky, Flat-Coated Retriever, Great Dane and Samoyed. In an emergency situation it can be difficult to recall all predisposed breeds but if a pure-breed dog presents with an acutely red, painful eye, and no other cause is clearly identified, glaucoma must always be considered and promptly excluded.

References and further reading

Bentley E, Miller PE, Murphy CJ, Schoster JV (1999) Combined cycloablation and gonioimplantation for treatment of glaucoma in dogs: 18 cases (1992–1998). *J Am Vet Med Assoc*, **215**, 1469–1472.

Miller PE, Schmidt GM, Vainisi SJ, Swanson JF, Herrman MK (2000) The efficacy of topical prophylactic antiglaucoma therapy in primary closed angle glaucoma in dogs: a multicentre clinical trial. *J Am Animal Hosp Assoc*, **36**, 431–438.

Miller PE, Struble C, Burke JA, Lee SS, Robinson MR (2010) Topical application of 0.005% latanoprost increases episcleral venous pressure in dogs. *Proc Am Coll Vet Ophthalmol, San Diego 2010, Vet Ophthalmol*, **13** (6), 407–423.

Sapienza J & van der Woerdt A (2005) Combined transscleral diode laser cyclophotocoagulation and Ahmed gonioimplantation in dogs with primary glaucoma: 51 cases (1996–2004). *Vet Ophthalmol*, **8**, 121–127.

See Appendix 2.

History

A 6-year-old male neutered Cocker Spaniel is presented with a six-week history of redness in the right eye. The dog has received routine vaccinations and anthelmintic treatment and is reportedly otherwise well.

Questions

1. Describe the abnormalities and pertinent normal features in Fig. 6.3a.
2. What differential diagnosis should be considered for this presentation?
3. What tests could you perform to make the diagnosis?

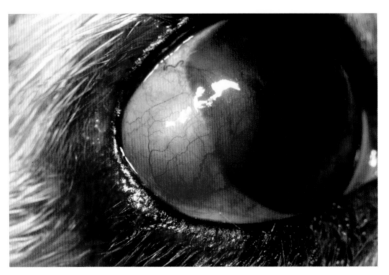

Fig. 6.3a

Answers

1. What the figure shows

Fig. 6.3a Right eye – there is a circular, raised lesion which is approximately 1 cm in diameter; it appears to involve the limbus and adjacent cornea, conjunctiva and sclera. The conjunctival vessels are hyperaemic and tortuous. The Purkinje images overlying the lesion are disrupted.

2. Differential diagnoses

Given the appearance of the right eye, the following conditions should be considered:

- **Nodular granulomatous episclerokeratitis (NGE)** NGE (or ocular nodular fasciitis) is an inflammatory condition which primarily involves the episclera, conjunctiva and cornea. The clinical appearance ranges from an irregular thickening to a pink, fleshy, discrete mass or nodule adjacent to or centred on the limbus; the dorsolateral quadrant is commonly affected. There is usually a superficial to mid-stromal vascular response in the adjacent cornea; the cornea may be oedematous and have lipid and mineral deposits. The TEL can be affected and appears hyperaemic, thickened and depigmented. Involvement of the eyelids and uveal tract has also been described. There is a predisposition for the Collie breeds, Cocker Spaniel, and the Shetland Sheepdog, but any breed can be affected. The condition may be unilateral or bilateral but is invariably bilateral in the Collie. A mixed inflammatory infiltrate composed predominantly of lymphocytes, plasma cells and histiocytes with a variable spindle cell component is seen on histopathology.
- **Neoplasia** Primary and secondary neoplasia can affect the region of the limbus in the dog. These include lymphoma (unilateral or bilateral white-to-pink corneal infiltrate), squamous cell carcinoma (raised pink mass with an irregular surface), amelanotic limbal melanoma (a smooth raised white-to-grey mass) and haemangioma/haemangiosarcoma (raised red mass).
- **Granulomatous episcleral disease** Localised episcleritis caused by trauma (foreign body, surgery), bacterial infection (e.g. *Mycobacterium* sp), parasitic infection (e.g. *Onchocerca* sp), protozoal infection (e.g. *Leishmania* sp), rickettsial infection (e.g. *Ehrlichia* sp), and fungal infection (e.g. *Blastomyces dermatitidis*). Diagnosis is made from biopsy and histopathology. The histopathological appearance of granulomatous episcleral disease differs from nodular episcleritis. By definition the inflammatory infiltrate is granulomatous and there are increased numbers of epithelioid macrophages and giant cells. Special stains may reveal infectious organisms and foreign material.
- **Systemic histiocytosis** Ocular signs are characterised by multiple masses involving the eyelid and episclera, exophthalmos, uveitis, retinal detachment, and glaucoma. Ocular disease occurs in conjunction with systemic signs which include anorexia, weight loss, depression and cutaneous nodules. Histiocytosis is considered to be an immunoregulatory disorder of the dermal dendritic cells. It is familial in the Bernese Mountain Dog but can occur in other breeds. Differentiation from malignant histiocytosis is aided by the lack of cellular atypia and immunohistochemical staining.

3. Appropriate diagnostic tests

- Ocular reflexes
  - Pupillary light reflex – direct and consensual positive OU
  - Dazzle reflex – positive OU
- Menace response – positive OU
- Examination with a focal light source – slit-lamp biomicroscopy reveals a vascular infiltrate which involves the corneal stroma in the right eye.
- Schirmer tear test – 18 mm/min OU
- Fluorescein dye – negative staining OU

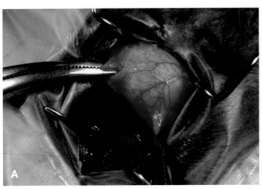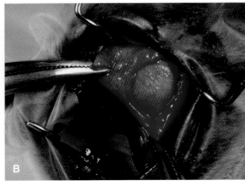

Fig. 6.3b (A) Artery forceps positioned onto the bulbar conjunctiva posterior to the limbus to faciliate maximum exposure of the lesion. (B) The conjunctiva is incised to expose the underlying episclera for biopsy.

- Tonometry – IOP 16 mmHg OU
- Gonioscopy – normal filtration angle OU; however it is not possible to assess the filtration angle beneath the raised lesion in the right eye.
- Laboratory tests – routine haematology, biochemistry and urine analysis are unremarkable.
- Histopathology – under general anaesthesia and with the aid of magnification, the conjunctiva overlying the lesion are incised to expose the underlying episcleral tissue (Fig. 6.3b). The abnormal tissue is excised and submitted for histopathology. Histopathology reveals a mixed inflammatory infiltrate in the episclera including lymphocytes, plasma cells, macrophages, and fibroblasts centred on the episclera. There is no evidence of infection, foreign material or neoplasia.

The remainder of the ophthalmic examination reveals no additional abnormalities and a general physical examination is unremarkable.

Diagnosis
Based on the information available, a diagnosis of nodular episcleritis in the right eye is made.

Treatment
Topical immunosuppression with 1% prednisolone acetate or 0.1% dexamethasone is the preferred initial therapy for nodular episcleritis. The frequency of treatment is typically q4–6 hours until the condition improves and the drug can then be tapered over several weeks. Recurrence is more common with bilateral disease. Topical therapy alone may be insufficient in some dogs with nodular episcleritis. Surgical excision or debulking, followed by strontium[90] therapy, cryotherapy or electrocautery usually facilitates prompt remission. An intralesional injection of a long-acting corticosteroid is also a useful adjunctive therapy. Systemic treatment with corticosteroids with or without azathioprine, and oxytetracycline with or without niacinamide, may also be considered in conjunction with the topical corticosteroid therapy. Systemic treatment can be tapered and eventually discontinued in some dogs.

In this dog remission is achieved after three months of 1% prednisolone acetate therapy (Fig. 6.3c) and maintenance therapy is continued once daily. Signs of recurrence develop one year later, i.e. conjunctival hyperaemia and increased vascularisation with a light tan discolouration of the adjacent cornea (Fig. 6.3d). Lipidosis also develops at the leading edge of the corneal pathology which is probably the result of chronic topical corticosteroid therapy in combination with the disease process itself. Topical treatment with 1% prednisolone acetate is re-started q6 hours to regain control of the disease and is subsequently tapered to q12 hours as the hyperaemia improves.

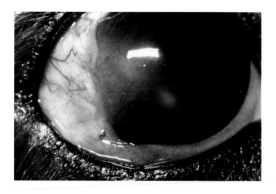

Fig. 6.3c Remission after three months of treatment, as indicated by reduced vascularisation, hyperaemia and thickening.

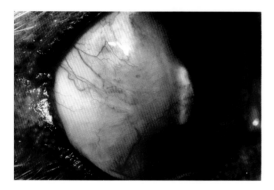

Fig. 6.3d Recurrence at one year appearing as an expanding area of increased conjunctival and episcleral hyperaemia and thickening, and vascularisation and tan discolouration of the adjacent cornea. Corneal lipidosis at the leading edge of the lesion is a result of chronic topical corticosteroid treatment as well as the disease process itself.

Prognosis

The prognosis for maintaining a non-inflamed and visual eye is excellent with early diagnosis, appropriate treatment and careful monitoring. Recurrence, however, is not uncommon. Inherently, the population of T and B lymphocytes differs between different forms of episcleritis, as demonstrated by immunohistochemical staining. This is of clinical relevance because lesions with a predominantly B-lymphocyte population are less likely to completely resolve and more likely to require long-term treatment to prevent recurrence.

Discussion

Episcleritis and scleritis are complex ocular conditions, not only because of the overlap in clinical signs but also because the nomenclature is highly variable in the human and veterinary fields. The most common clinical forms in dogs are nodular and diffuse episcleritis, with the syndrome in the Collie breed considered a separate condition by some authors. Synonyms for nodular episcleritis include nodular granulomatous episcleritis (NGE), pseudotumour, fibrous histiocytoma, nodular fasciitis, proliferative keratoconjunctivitis, limbal granulomas and Collie granulomas. Nodular and diffuse episcleritis are considered to be a primary condition; secondary forms of episcleritis are caused by trauma or infection. Scleritis is a more severe disease in the dog and can be necrotizing or non-necrotizing. The clinical appearance of diffuse episcleritis (as opposed to nodular episcleritis), and both forms of scleritis (necrotising and non-necrotising) is similar and a specific diagnosis can only be made with histopathology. The extent and degree of inflammation associated with scleritis is more severe to that seen in dogs with episcleritis. Extension of inflammation into the adjacent uveal tract can occur, particularly within the posterior segment, resulting in uveitis and retinal detachment. Scleritis is also presumed to be an immune-mediated disease and is treated with immunosuppressive drugs. The prognosis for scleritis is very guarded, in contrast to diffuse episcleritis for which the prognosis is good with appropriate management.

References and further reading

Grahn BH & Sandmeyer LS (2008) Canine episcleritis, nodular episclerokeratitis, scleritis and necrotic scleritis. *Vet Clin North Am: Small Animal Pract*, **38** (2), 291–308.

See Appendix 2.

CHAPTER 7

The Opaque Eye

Introduction

The retina relies on the optical clarity of the visual axis to receive a clear and precise image. Opacity may be the result of multiple single ocular defects, the extent of which can be variable. With experience and a thorough ocular examination, the exact location of an opacity in the eye can readily be determined and a list of possible causes identified.

Small Animal Ophthalmology: What's Your Diagnosis? First Edition. Heidi Featherstone, Elaine Holt.
© 2011 by Heidi Featherstone and Elaine Holt. Published 2011 by Blackwell Publishing Ltd.

History

A 5-year-old male neutered terrier-cross dog is presented with a 10-day history of progressive cloudiness in both eyes and bumping into furniture. The dog was diagnosed with diabetes mellitus three months previously and is considered to be clinically stable on insulin therapy.

Questions

1. Describe the abnormalities and pertinent normal features in Figs. 7.1a and b.
2. What differential diagnoses should be considered for this presentation?
3. What tests could you perform to make the diagnosis?

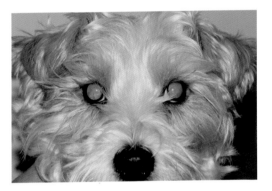

Fig. 7.1a Reproduced with permission from J Mould.

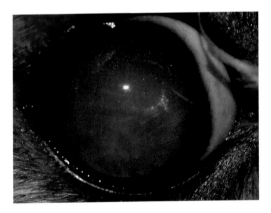

Fig. 7.1b Reproduced with permission from J Mould.

Answers

1. What the figures show

Fig. 7.1a Both eyes have received tropicamide to dilate the pupil – the left and right eyes are similar. There is leukocoria (white pupil) and the tapetal reflection is absent.

Fig. 7.1b Right eye – there is a crystalline, white appearance to the lens. The ocular surface is lustrous.

2. Differential diagnoses

Given the appearance of the both eyes, the following conditions should be considered:

- **Lens abnormalities**
  - **Cataract** The term cataract describes any opacity of the lens. Cataracts can be classified in several ways including by the age of onset, degree of maturity, location within the lens, appearance (shape and form), and cause. The most common types of cataract in the dog are heritable, senile, diabetic and those secondary to retinal disease such as progressive retinal atrophy (*Ch. 11, case 1*).
  - **Nuclear sclerosis (lenticular sclerosis)** This is a normal age-related change which involves compression of the lens nucleus by the expansion of the outer cortex from the continuous addition of new lens fibres throughout life. This process of compression begins around six to seven years in the dog. The change in the optical properties of the compressed nucleus causes light scattering, which imparts a whitish blue or opalescent appearance to the lens when viewed with diffuse illumination. Affected eyes still have vision and, with experience, it is still possible to examine the fundus. In the human lens, this process starts in the fourth decade of life and results in presbyopia – a reduction in the ability of the lens to focus on near objects. Nuclear sclerosis can be differentiated from a cataract using retro-illumination from the tapetum. A tapetal reflection is present with nuclear sclerosis, but is partially obscured by an immature cataract and is absent with a mature cataract (Fig. 7.1c).
  - **Persistent hyperplastic primary vitreous (PHPV)** PHPV appears as a white or fibrovascular plaque posterior to the pupil. It is a congenital abnormality characterised by a retrolental mass formed by remnants of the hyaloid system and the tunica vasculosa lentis. PHPV is a heritable condition in the Doberman Pinscher and the Staffordshire Bull Terrier but can occur as a spontaneous disorder in any breed. It is usually unilateral.

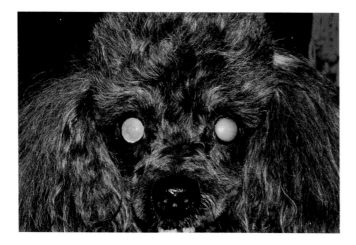

Fig. 7.1c A 10-year-old Miniature Poodle with a mature cataract in the left eye and nuclear sclerosis in the right eye. Reproduced with permission from J Mould.

- **Opacities in the vitreous humour**
  - ○ **Asteroid hyalosis** This is a degenerative change of the vitreous humour which is manifested by whitish spherical bodies containing calcium and phospholipids suspended within the vitreous. These bodies move slightly with eye movement and are a feature of advanced age and ciliary body neoplasia. Affected eyes are visual (assuming no concurrent pathology) and fundic examination is possible.
  - ○ **Synchysis scintillans** This term describes refractile particles of cholesterol within a more or less liquefied vitreous humour (vitreal syneresis). These particles usually disperse and then gravitate with eye movement. Synchysis scintillans is also a degenerative change; it is a feature of advanced age and can follow episodes of intraocular inflammation. Fundic examination is usually still possible.
- **Retinal detachment** Separation of the neurosensory retina from the underlying retinal pigment epithelium results in anterior displacement of the detached retina. This appears as a grey sheet containing blood vessels behind the pupil.
- **Intraocular neoplasia** Neoplasia within the posterior segment may manifest as leukocoria, e.g. ciliary body tumour (adenoma/adenocarcinoma), medullo-epithelioma or amelanotic melanoma.

3. Appropriate diagnostic tests

- Ocular reflexes
  - ○ Pupillary light reflex – direct and consensual positive OU
  - ○ Dazzle reflex – positive OU
- Vision testing
  - ○ Menace response – negative OU
  - ○ Visual placing and tracking reflexes – negative OU
  - ○ Maze test (obstacle course) – this dog is unable to navigate large objects in photopic conditions.

These results suggest that this dog is blind but that retinal and optic nerve function is present in both eyes.

- Examination with a focal light source – this reveals normal depth and transparency of the anterior chamber in both eyes.
- Tonometry – IOP 12 mmHg OU
- Gonioscopy – normal filtration angle OU (*Ch. 6, case 2, Diagram 6.2*)
- B-mode ocular ultrasound – ultrasound is helpful in animals with cataract to assess the posterior region of the lens and the posterior segment of the eye. Rapidly forming cataract can result in an increase in lens volume from absorption of aqueous humour; this is known as intumescence. Rapid intumescence may cause rupture of the lens capsule (most frequently the thinner posterior lens capsule) and expulsion of cortical material. Diabetic cataracts in dogs form rapidly and an increase in lens volume can be readily assessed with ultrasound by measuring the axial length of the lens. This is the distance from the centre of the anterior lens capsule to the centre of posterior lens capsule (Fig. 7.1d, B). A posterior lens capsule rupture is seen as a focal hyperechoic area at the junction of the posterior lens and the adjacent anterior vitreous, or as a break in the normal contour of the posterior lens. Partial or total retinal detachment, vitreal degeneration and a persistent hyaloid artery are also detectable on ocular ultrasound, all of which might affect the success of cataract surgery.

In both eyes the ultrasound scan reveals a hyperechoic lens consistent with cataract (Fig. 7.1d, A) and an axial lens length of 7.5 mm (within normal limits).

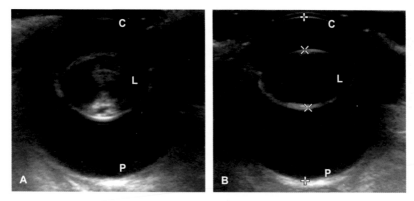

Fig. 7.1d B-mode ultrasound scans. (A) Axial regions of the anterior and posterior cortices of the lens in this dog are hyperechoic, consistent with cataract. (B) Normal eye from a dog without cataract – the convex anterior and posterior aspects of the hypoechoic lens are represented by hyperechoic curvilinear lines (X). C, cornea; L, lens; P, posterior outline of globe.

- Electroretinography (ERG) – ERG is a means by which retinal function can be assessed when the fundus cannot be observed with ophthalmoscopy. Assessment of retinal function is important prior to cataract surgery because a cataract can develop secondary to retinal degeneration (*Ch. 11, case 1*) and some breeds are predisposed to both heritable cataract and heritable retinal degeneration. Cataract surgery is contraindicated in an eye with poor or absent retinal function.

  In this dog, ERG reveals that the b-wave amplitude and latency are within the normal range for both eyes. This is consistent with satisfactory retinal function in both eyes.
- Laboratory tests – results of routine haematology, biochemistry, and urine analysis are consistent with clinically controlled diabetes mellitus.

The remainder of the ophthalmic examination reveals no additional abnormalities; a general physical examination, including blood pressure assessment, is unremarkable.

Diagnosis
Based on the information available, a diagnosis of a mature diabetic cataract is made in both eyes.

Treatment
The two most important consequences of cataracts are impaired vision or blindness and lens-induced uveitis (LIU). Both should be assessed when considering treatment. Phacoemulsification is the standard technique for cataract extraction in man and animals. It involves the use of high-frequency ultrasonic vibrations to break up the lens, irrigation to maintain a formed anterior chamber and aspiration to remove the lens fragments. The procedure is performed through a small corneal incision (typically <3 mm). Phacoemulsification is a highly specialised intraocular surgical procedure which requires microsurgical instrumentation, an operating microscope, neuromuscular blockade anaesthesia and appropriate training. Where possible, an artificial intraocular lens is placed into the lens capsular bag following removal of the cataract. LIU (phacolytic uveitis) occurs to some degree with most cataracts but is most marked in rapidly developing cataracts, especially those caused by diabetes mellitus and trauma. Clinical signs include conjunctival hyperaemia, darkening of the iris, and hypotony (Fig. 7.1e). LIU should ideally be managed prior to surgery with topical and/or systemic anti-inflammatory therapy to reduce the risk of long-term

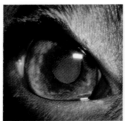
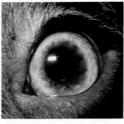

Fig. 7.1e Lens-induced uveitis causes darkening of the iris in the right eye of a young Labrador; the left eye is normal.

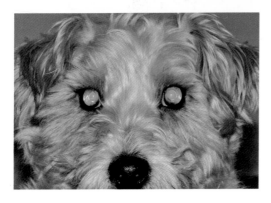

Fig. 7.1f Two weeks following routine cataract extraction by phacoemulsification and artificial intraocular lens implantation. Note the clarity of the visual axes compared to that in Fig. 7.1a and the restored tapetal reflection in both eyes. Reproduced with permission from J Mould.

postoperative complications. If cataract surgery is not elected, the patient should be monitored on a regular basis for complications secondary to LIU, e.g. glaucoma, lens luxation and retinal detachment. Cataract surgery is an elective procedure as many dogs will adapt well to being blind.

As the clinical signs of LIU are limited to mild hypotony in this dog, both eyes receive topical 0.5% ketorolac trometamol q12 hours prior to surgery. Bilateral phacoemulsification and artificial lens implantation is performed and results in improved postoperative vision. (Fig. 7.1f).

Prognosis
The prognosis for vision following routine cataract extraction by phacoemulsifcation is very good, with an average short-term success rate of 90–95% in dogs (Wilkie & Colitz, 2007). Diligent long-term postoperative monitoring is essential as complications may occur months to years after surgery, e.g. posterior capsular opacity, uveitis, glaucoma and retinal detachment.

Discussion
Diabetic cataracts are very common in dogs – 50% of dogs develop cataract within 170 days of diagnosis and 80% within 470 days (Beam *et al.*, 1999). Hyperglycaemia leads to an accumulation of glucose in the lens, which alters the normal lens metabolism. The metabolism of glucose in the lens is primarily through anaerobic glycolysis (Embden-Meyerhof pathway). In dogs with hyperglycaemia this pathway is saturated and excess glucose is converted to sorbitol by the enzyme aldose reductase. Sorbitol accumulates in the lens and, because it is a large sugar molecule, cannot readily diffuse through the lens capsule. This creates an osmotic gradient and aqueous humour is rapidly imbibed causing swelling of lens fibres; as a result the lens becomes opaque. Diabetic cataracts are usually bilateral and symmetrical; they often form very rapidly (sometimes within a few days to a week), and are characterised by moderate to marked LIU. Intumescence of the lens and spontaneous lens rupture can occur. Signs of anterior lens capsule rupture are usually be detected by examination with a focal light source or with slit-lamp biomicroscopy, whereas signs of posterior

lens capsule rupture may only be detected with preoperative ocular ultrasonography. In general, diabetic cataracts benefit from early surgery, as long as the patient is sufficiently stable to undergo general anaesthesia safely.

References and further reading

Beam S, Correa MT, Davidson MG (1999) A retrospective-cohort study on the development of cataracts in dogs with diabetes mellitus: 200 cases. *Vet Ophthalmol* **2**, 169–172.

Wilkie DA & Colitz CMH (2007) Surgery of the canine lens. In: *Veterinary Ophthalmology*, Ed., KN Gelatt, 4th edn, Blackwell Publishing, Iowa, USA, p 905.

See Appendix 2.

History

A 1-year-old female neutered domestic shorthaired cat is presented with a two-week history of lethargy and cloudiness in the left eye. The cat lives in a multi-cat household; all the cats have been routinely vaccinated, have received regular anthelmintic treatment and are indoor/outdoor cats.

Questions

1. Describe the abnormalities and pertinent normal features in Figs. 7.2a and b.
2. What differential diagnoses should be considered for this presentation?
3. What tests could you perform to make the diagnosis?

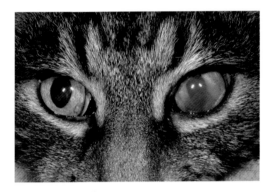

Fig. 7.2a

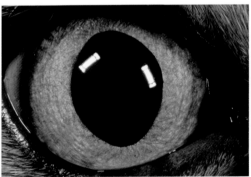

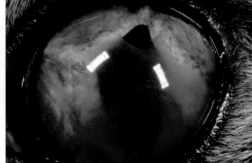

Fig. 7.2b

Answers

1. What the figures show
Fig. 7.2a The right eye is normal. Left eye – there is pink and grey opacification in front of the pupil.
Fig. 7.2b Left eye – there is a subtle diffuse corneal haze and a large clot of fibrin and blood in the anterior chamber. The iris is darker in areas and seems distorted; dyscoria is present. There is a relative anisocoria (OS < OD).

2. Differential diagnoses
Given the appearance of the left eye, the clinical diagnosis is anterior uveitis. The following causes for uveitis should be considered:
- **Infection**
  - ○ **Viral** The following agents can cause uveitis in the cat: feline immunodeficiency virus (FIV), feline infectious peritonitis (FIP), feline leukemia virus (FeLV) and feline herpesvirus-1 (FHV-1). Although both anterior and posterior uveitis can occur with all these viruses, there are specific characteristics associated with each, e.g. pars planitis with FIV; keratic precipitates, fibrin in the anterior chamber, and pyogranulomatous chorioretinitis with FIP; and white-to-pink uveal masses (lymphoma) with FeLV.
  - ○ **Protozoal** Both anterior and posterior uveitis are well documented features of cats with systemic signs of toxoplasmosis. However the role of toxoplasmosis in healthy cats with uveitis, especially anterior uveitis alone, is controversial (Davidson & English, 1998). A definitive diagnosis of toxoplasmosis can only be confirmed by demonstration of *Toxoplasma gondii* on histopathology. A presumptive diagnosis of ocular toxoplasmosis is based on clinical signs, response to antitoxoplasmic therapy and supportive diagnostic tests, i.e. high IgM titre, rising IgG titre, IgM C-value >1, positive PCR results.
  - ○ **Bacterial** Bacterial infection can occur with penetrating trauma, septicaemia, and systemic infection with, e.g. *Bartonella henselae, Mycobacterium* sp, and *Leishmania* sp. Although *Bartonella henselae* has been considered to be a causal agent of feline uveitis, the presence or magnitude of serum antibodies to *Bartonella* sp cannot be used alone to document ocular bartonellosis (Fontenelle *et al.*, 2008).
  - ○ **Fungal** Granulomatous anterior uveitis, often with concurrent chorioretinitis, can occur with *Cryptococcus neoformans, Histoplasma capsulatum, Coccidioides immitis, Blastomyces dermatidis* and *Candida* sp.
  - ○ **Parasitic (ophthalmomyiasis)** Anterior and posterior uveitis occur rarely, e.g. larva of *Cuterebra* sp.
- **Lymphoplasmacytic uveitis** This is considered to be an immune-mediated process and is characterised by unilateral or bilateral chronic disease in middle-aged to older cats. Lymphoplasmacytic uveitis often causes secondary glaucoma which can necessitate enucleation. The diagnosis is made by exclusion.
- **Neoplasia** Both primary and secondary neoplasia may cause uveitis. Primary intraocular neoplasia in the cat includes diffuse iris melanoma (*Ch. 9, case 3*), post-traumatic sarcoma and ciliary epithelial tumours. All can cause a colour change within the eye in conjunction with uveitis. The most common secondary uveal neoplasm in the cat is lymphoma which can appear in two forms – a focal iridal mass or anterior uveitis. Metastatic disease and local invasion of extraocular tumours can also result in uveitis.
- **Trauma** Penetrating or blunt trauma can cause acute onset uveitis with pain and hyphaema.
- **Corneal ulcer** Corneal stimulation incites an axonal reflex mediated by substance P and results in iridocyclospasm and subsequent miosis (*Ch. 10, case 1*).

- **Lens-induced uveitis** This form of uveitis can develop with rapidly forming traumatic cataracts (phacoclastic uveitis) or hypermature cataracts (phacolytic uveitis). Lens luxation may also cause uveitis. Lens-induced uveitis in the cat is generally less intense than its counterpart in the dog (*case 1, this chapter*).
- **Vascular disease** Systemic hypertension may cause anterior segment signs that mimic anterior uveitis (*Ch. 1, case 1*). Other less common causes of vascular disease include polycythaemia and hyperviscosity syndrome.

3. Appropriate diagnostic tests

- Ocular reflexes
  - Pupillary light reflex – positive direct and consensual OU. There is reduced mobility of the left pupil.
  - Dazzle reflex – positive OU
- Menace response – negative OS and positive OD

In this cat, these results suggest that there is a visual deficit in the left eye but that retinal and optic nerve function are still present.

- Examination with a focal light source – in the left eye, slit-lamp biomicroscopy reveals a slight increase in the corneal thickness (because of oedema), aqueous flare, hyperaemia of the iridal vasculature, multifocal posterior synechiae and inflammatory cells on the anterior lens capsule manifested by a dust-like covering on the surface of the lens. The posterior synechiae most likely account for the reduced pupil mobility.
- Schirmer tear test – 10 mm/min OU
- Fluorescein dye – negative staining OU
- Tonometry – IOP 14 mmHg OS, 22 mmHg OD

The remainder of the ophthalmic examination reveals no abnormalities and a general physical examination is unremarkable.

Further diagnostic tests

- B-mode ocular ultrasound – this reveals thickening of the iris and hyperechoic material in the anterior chamber, consistent with a fibrin clot. The posterior segment is unremarkable.
- Laboratory tests – routine haematology, biochemistry, urine analysis and serological tests for common infectious agents for a cat in north Europe (*Toxoplasma gondii*, FIV, FeLV and FIP) are performed. This is an initial screening examination with a view to selecting more specific tests if indicated. The cat is lymphopaenic, leukopaenic and positive for both FIV and FeLV.
- Thoracic radiography and abdominal ultrasound – the results are unremarkable.
- Anterior chamber paracentesis – aqueous humour can be sampled for cytology, bacteriology, antibody titres (to determine the C-value) and PCR assay for infectious agents. Aqueous paracentesis is usually performed under sedation or general anaesthesia and is not without risk – appropriate training to perform this procedure is essential (Fig. 7.2c). The procedure should be reserved for selected cases as it can exacerbate uveitis and results may be unrewarding. Aqueous paracentesis is probably best indicated when there is a strong clinical suspicion of lymphoma, or when C-values might be helpful. It is not indicated in this cat because of the positive FIV and FeLV status.

Aqueous humour titre levels can be compared to those in the serum to determine whether there is local antibody production against a specific antigen. A Goldmann-Witmer coefficient, or C-value, of >1 indicates local antibody production. The formula to determine the C-value is: (antibody specific Ig in aqueous humour/antibody specific Ig in serum) × (total Ig in aqueous humour/total Ig in serum)

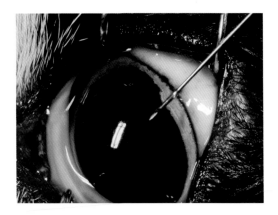

Fig. 7.2c Aqueous humour paracentesis performed on a cat under general anaesthesia. After preparation of the ocular surface with dilute povidone-iodine solution a topical anaesthetic is applied. A 25-gauge needle is inserted through the limbus at an oblique angle and advanced; contact with the corneal endothelium, iris and lens should be avoided. A volume of 0.1–0.25 ml aqueous humour can be slowly aspirated.

Diagnosis

Based on the information available, a diagnosis of anterior uveitis in the left eye is made, this is most probably the result of a combined infection with FIV and FeLV.

Treatment

Non-specific treatment of feline anterior uveitis consists primarily of topical mydriatic/cycloplegic and anti-inflammatory drugs. Atropine is a potent mydriatic and cycloplegic agent, and will relieve ciliary body spasm as well as reduce the risk of posterior synechiae formation. The frequency of application should be titrated to achieve and maintain mydriasis – this is typically q12–24 hours in the cat but depends on the degree of uveitis.

> Atropine is a parasympatholytic agent which reduces salivation. However, atropine is bitter and may cause profuse salivation after topical administration of eye drops as the solution formulation travels rapidly down the nasolacrimal duct to the oral cavity. This effect can be especially marked in cats, although it may occur in some dogs. An ointment formulation is therefore preferable in the cat to reduce passage of the drug through the nasolacrimal duct.

The topical anti-inflammatory agents of choice are 1% prednisolone acetate or 0.1% dexamethasone. The frequency of administration will depend on the severity of the uveitis (q6–12 hours) and the drug should be tapered as the clinical signs improve. Although systemic anti-inflammatory therapy is indicated if the posterior segment is involved, NSAIDs are preferable to corticosteroids if the underlying disease process is thought to be infectious, e.g. generalised toxoplasmosis. Persisting fibrin can lead to the formation of posterior synechiae and secondary glaucoma. If fibrin in the anterior chamber persists despite anti-inflammatory therapy, an intracameral injection of tissue plasminogen activator (TPA) can be administered. TPA is most effective at dissolving a fibrin clot that has been present for <72 hours but may be effective for up to 10 days.

Topical therapy in this cat includes 1% atropine ointment once daily for three days then twice weekly for two weeks, in conjunction with 1% prednisolone acetate q6 hours for one week, then tapered over four weeks to a maintenance dose of q24 hours.

Prognosis

The prognosis for a visual, normotensive eye following an episode of feline uveitis is guarded. Posterior synechiae, iris bombé (*Ch. 9, case 4*), the formation of pre-iridal fibrovascular membranes (*Ch. 1, case 1*), cataract and glaucoma can all result from severe and/or protracted uveitis. Glaucoma is common, occurring in 46% of cats either at the time of the initial diagnosis of uveitis or at follow-up examinations (Davidson *et al.*, 1991). Cataracts are also a common complication, occurring in 36% of cats with idiopathic lymphoplasmacytic uveitis (Gemensky *et al.*, 1996). These authors also found that idiopathic uveitis and uveitis secondary to FIV were more responsive to treatment (56%) than uveitis associated with other systemic disease (33%).

Discussion

The clinical signs of uveitis in the cat are often more subtle than in the dog, and cats often present with advanced disease or even secondary glaucoma. Pain may be absent or mild and conjunctival hyperaemia is difficult to observe (conjunctiva is less visible than in the dog). However iris discoloration because of vascular hyperaemia or infiltration by inflammatory or neoplastic cells is readily observed in the cat because the iris is generally a light colour. Keratic precipitates are also more common than in the dog and are readily observed against a light-coloured iris. In summary, a dog with anterior uveitis is more likely to present with acute discomfort or pain, whereas a cat with anterior uveitis is more likely to present with a change in the appearance of the eye.

References and further reading

Davidson MG & English RV (1998) Feline ocular toxoplasmosis. *Vet Ophthalmol* **1**, 71–80.

Davidson MG, Nasisse MP, English RV, Wilcock BP, Jamieson VE (1991) Feline anterior uveitis: a study of 53 cases. *J Am Animal Hosp Assoc*, **27** (1), 77–83.

Fontenelle JP, Powell CP, Hill AE, Radecki SV, Lappin MR (2008) Prevalence of serum antibodies against *Bartonella* sp in the serum of cats with and without uveitis. *J Feline Med Surg* **10**, 41–46.

Gemensky A, Lorimer D, Blanchard D (1996) A retrospective study of 45 cases. *Proc Am Coll Vet Ophthalmol*, **27**:19.

Maggs DJ, Lappin MR, Nasisse MP (1999) Detection of feline herpesvirus-specific antibodies and DNA in aqueous humour from cats with or without uveitis. *Am J Vet Res*, **60** (8), 932–936.

See Appendix 2.

History

A 9-year-old female neutered Miniature Schnauzer is presented because of sudden onset cloudiness in the right eye shortly after eating buttered toast. The dog underwent bilateral cataract surgery six weeks previously, and has received routine vaccinations and regular anthelmintic treatment.

Questions

1. Describe the abnormalities and pertinent normal features in Figs. 7.3a and b.
2. What differential diagnoses should be considered for this presentation?
3. What tests could you perform to make the diagnosis?

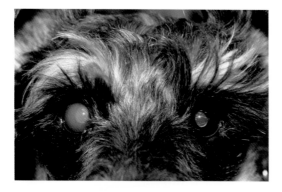

Fig. 7.3a

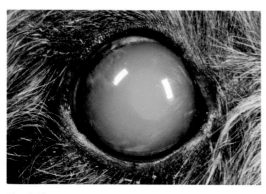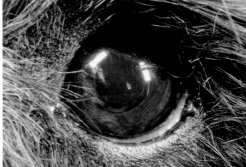

Fig. 7.3b

Answers

1. What the figures show
Fig. 7.3a Left eye – there is a refractile structure within the pupil and a good tapetal reflection. Right eye – there is diffuse cloudiness which appears to be anterior to the iris; a tapetal reflection is still visible.

Fig. 7.3b Both eyes are shown. There is anisocoria (OD < OS) and the Purkinje images are normal. Left eye – the iris is dark and mottled and the round refractile structure within the pupil is consistent with the edge of the optic of an artificial intraocular lens. Right eye – the conjunctiva is pigmented on the dorsal and lateral aspects of the eye, a common and normal finding. There is a notable lack of redness and discharge.

2. Differential diagnoses
Given the history and the appearance of the right eye, the following conditions should be considered:

- **Anterior chamber opacity**
  - **Lipid aqueous (aqueous lipaemia)** A transient and poorly understood phenomenon that results from a breakdown of the blood-aqueous barrier in the presence of hyperlipidaemia; the aqueous humour is opaque because of the presence of lipid. Lipid aqueous can occur spontaneously, or in association with uveitis, e.g. following intraocular surgery.
  - **Anterior lens luxation (with cataract)** Anterior luxation of a cataractous lens results in opacification of the anterior chamber. This combination is most often seen with hypermature and senile cataract because of degenerative changes within the lens zonules. Alternatively a luxated lens will undergo cataractous change which can progress to complete opacification with time (*Ch. 5, case 3*).
  - **Aqueous flare** Breakdown of the blood-aqueous barrier results in protein and sometimes cells in the aqueous humour. Aqueous flare is best seen as a continuous light reflection throughout the anterior chamber. Particles suspended in the aqueous humour scatter light to produce the effect known as the Tyndall phenomenon. It is considered to be pathognomonic for anterior uveitis. The degree of aqueous flare can be subjectively graded as 1+ if barely detectable through to 4+ for the most intense flare, e.g. coagulated aqueous and fibrin which obscures iris and lens detail.
  - **Fibrinous aqueous (plasmoid aqueous)** This occurs if protein levels in the aqueous humour increase to approximate that of normal plasma. This is most commonly seen with acute, severe anterior uveitis. Fibrin clots form in the anterior chamber if fibrinous exudation is severe.
- **Corneal opacity** Corneal transparency is a result of the precise arrangement of collagen fibrils within the stroma which minimises the scattering of light rays, the absence of blood vessels and pigment, and a low water content.
  - **Corneal oedema** Hydration of the corneal stroma appears as a characteristic dull blue-grey opacity because of the scattering of light rays. Causes of corneal oedema include age-related corneal endothelial degeneration, corneal endothelial dystrophy, corneal endothelial damage (secondary to glaucoma, uveitis, anterior lens luxation, intraocular surgery, toxins), corneal ulceration and endotheliitis (*Ch. 8, case 1*).
  - **Crystalline corneal opacities** These arise from lipid and mineral deposition, e.g. lipid keratopathy (corneal lipidosis), corneal dystrophy, corneal degeneration, and calcific band keratopathy (*Ch. 8, case 2*).
  - **Corneal scarring** During stromal healing, new collagen fibres are laid down in a disorganised arrangement which causes scattering of light rays and corneal opacity. Corneal scars may be focal or generalised.

3. Appropriate diagnostic tests

- Ocular reflexes
  - Pupillary light reflex – direct and consensual positive OU
  - Dazzle reflex – positive OU
- Menace response – positive OU
- Examination with a focal light source – this reveals that an artificial intraocular lens is present in both eyes. Light directed at an oblique angle reveals that the cloudiness in the right eye appears to be evenly distributed throughout the anterior chamber; slit-lamp biomicroscopy confirms that the cloudiness is restricted to the anterior chamber and does not involve the cornea.
- Ophthalmoscopy – fundic examination is normal OU
- Schirmer tear test – 17 mm/min OU
- Fluorescein dye – negative staining OU
- Tonometry – IOP 16 mmHg OS, 7 mmHg OD
- Laboratory tests – routine haematology, biochemistry (including serum cholesterol and triglycerides), urine analysis, and tests for thyroid function are performed. The blood sample is grossly lipaemic (Fig. 7.3c) and the biochemistry results are consistent with post-prandial hyperlipidaemia.

Diagnosis

Based on the information available, a diagnosis of a lipid aqueous and anterior uveitis in the right eye is made.

Treatment

The treatment of anterior uveitis is thought to hasten the clearing of the lipid-laden aqueous humour, although this may also happen spontaneously. Treatment comprises topical anti-inflammatory therapy in conjunction with a low-fat diet. A topical corticosteroid (1% prednisolone acetate) or a NSAID (e.g. 0.5% ketorolac trometamol) is appropriate. Treatment of the underlying condition, if identified, is also indicated.

Prognosis

Lipid usually clears from the aqueous humour within 48–72 hours and so the prognosis for optical clarity is good. However, recurrence is possible if systemic hyperlipidaemia persists.

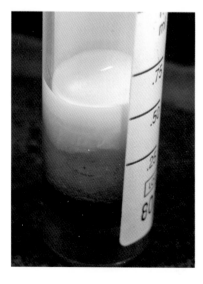

Fig. 7.3c Lipaemic serum.

Discussion

The development of lipid aqueous results from concurrent hyperlipidaemia. Transient hyperlipidaemia follows the ingestion of a meal (post-prandial hyperlipidaemia) and is normal. Primary hyperlipidaemia is uncommon in dogs but has been reported most frequently in the Miniature Schnauzer. Hyperlipidaemia as a result of diabetes mellitus, hypothyroidism, pancreatitis, hyper-adrenocorticism, nephrotic syndrome, and hepatic disease is more common.

A causal relationship between uveitis and hyperlipidaemia has been suggested. The blood-aqueous barrier prevents large particles, including lipoproteins, from entering the aqueous humour. However, following the breakdown of the blood-aqueous barrier in uveitis, lipid, protein and cells can pass freely into the aqueous humour. Lipid aqueous is most often seen following cataract surgery in dogs with diabetes mellitus or in dogs with uveitis prior to surgery. Lipid aqueous also occurs spontaneously in eyes without uveitis, suggesting that lipids can incite inflammation.

The importance of taking a detailed history is highlighted by this case. The Miniature Schnauzer is predisposed to primary hyperlipidaemia, diabetes mellitus and portosystemic shunts, all of which can cause hyperlipidaemia and lipid aqueous. Specific tests are not performed in this dog because of the known history of recent cataract surgery and the ingestion of a high fat meal prior to the onset of the problem.

Further reading

See Appendix 2.

CHAPTER 8

Corneal Opacities

Introduction

The main function of the cornea is the refraction of light. The transparency of the cornea is maintained by the parallel arrangement of stromal collagen fibres and by the corneal epithelium and endothelium, which play a critical role in keeping the cornea in a constant state of relative dehydration. The hallmark of corneal disease is opacity and these opacities vary in size and colour. White opacities (e.g. lipid, fibrosis) are easier to see than brown opacities (e.g. melanin), which may go unnoticed if viewed against the background of a dark iris. With experience and careful examination the location and exact colour of a corneal opacity can be determined, and a list of possible causes identified.

Small Animal Ophthalmology: What's Your Diagnosis? First Edition. Heidi Featherstone, Elaine Holt.
© 2011 by Heidi Featherstone and Elaine Holt. Published 2011 by Blackwell Publishing Ltd.

CASE STUDY 1

History

A 12-year-old female neutered English Springer Spaniel is presented with a six-month history of progressive cloudiness in both eyes. The owner has not observed any evidence of ocular discomfort but became concerned when the dog's vision seemed impaired and the surface of the right eye began to bulge. The dog has received routine vaccinations and regular anthelmintic treatment and is reported to be otherwise well.

Questions

1. Describe the abnormalities and pertinent normal features in Figs. 8.1a, b and c.
2. What differential diagnoses should be considered for this presentation?
3. What tests could you perform to make the diagnosis?

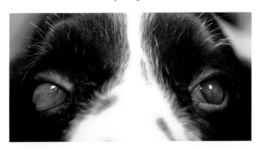

Fig. 8.1a

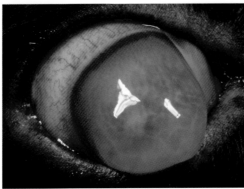

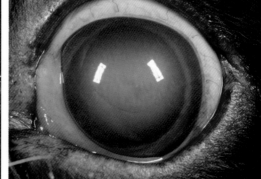

Fig. 8.1b

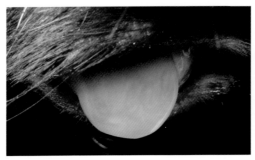

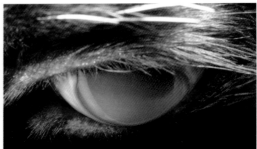

Fig. 8.1c

Answers

1. What the figures show

Fig. 8.1a Both eyes – the ocular surface is opaque; the TEL is non-pigmented, a normal variation in the dog. Right eye – there is an irregular contour to the ocular surface, which seems to protrude. There is epiphora and prominence of the TEL.

Fig. 8.1b Left eye – there is a seromucoid discharge at the medial canthus, mild conjunctival hyperaemia and normal Purkinje images. There is a mild diffuse corneal opacity involving approximately 70% of the cornea. The pupil is moderately dilated and the visible area of iris appears normal. Right eye – there is moderate conjunctival hyperaemia, a peri-limbal band of corneal vascularisation and distorted Purkinje images. The cornea is opaque, has an irregular contour and protrudes; there are multiple areas of lucency within the axial cornea. Intraocular structures are not visible.

Fig. 8.1c Aerial view. Left eye – the convex contour of the corneal surface is unremarkable; the anterior chamber is normal with respect to depth and clarity. Right eye – there is pronounced corneal convexity.

> Corneal transparency is a result of the precise arrangement of collagen fibrils, the relative dehydration of the stroma, and the absence of blood vessels.

2. Differential diagnoses

Given the appearance of the corneal opacification, the clinical diagnosis is bilateral corneal oedema. The following conditions should be considered:

- **Age-related corneal endothelial degeneration** This is a disease of spontaneous, progressive corneal oedema in geriatric dogs, resulting from an age-related decrease in corneal endothelial cell density. The normal corneal endothelial cell density in a young dog is approximately 3000 cells/mm^2. When this cell density decreases to between 800 and 500 cells/mm^2, the endothelial pump mechanism fails to maintain normal corneal dehydration – this is known as corneal decompensation. The corneal oedema that results has a bluish-white appearance and there is an initial, notable absence of conjunctival hyperaemia or corneal vascularisation. The oedema progresses slowly, over months to years, and although it may eventually cause visual impairment, most dogs retain an acceptable level of guidance vision. In more advanced cases, epithelial bullae result from the accumulation of fluid within the stroma. Ocular discomfort arises when focal corneal ulcers develop following rupture of the corneal bullae. Bilateral involvement is usually asymmetrical, as in this dog.
- **Corneal endothelial dystrophy** This refers to spontaneous, progressive corneal oedema resulting from dystrophic corneal endothelial cells. Although the number of endothelial cells is within normal limits, cell function is impaired because of abnormal development. This disease is most prevalent in the Boston Terrier, Chihuahua and Dachshund, although it has been reported in other breeds at different ages.
- **Non-specific corneal endothelial damage** This can be secondary to a variety of mechanisms including:
  - **Glaucoma** Diffuse corneal oedema develops when raised IOP impairs the function of the corneal endothelial pump mechanism. Increased hydration of the stroma results and leads to a distortion of the precise arrangement of the collagen fibres. Corneal oedema is typically seen when IOP is >40 mmHg.

- ○ **Uveitis** Inflammatory mediators cause increased corneal endothelial permeability and malfunction of the endothelial pump mechanism.
- ○ **Anterior lens luxation** Physical contact between the anterior surface of the lens and the corneal endothelium frequently causes focal (subaxial) corneal oedema in an eye with anterior lens luxation (*Ch. 5, case 3*). Secondary glaucoma and uveitis usually results in diffuse rather than focal oedema.
- ○ **Intraocular surgery** Mechanical trauma to the corneal endothelium from instruments, manipulation of the lens and intraocular irrigating solutions can cause corneal oedema.
- ○ **Toxins** Bilateral corneal oedema can occur with systemic drugs, e.g. chlorpromazine, tocainide and lortalamine.
- **Corneal ulcer** Localised oedema develops when the hydrophobic corneal epithelial barrier is disrupted or absent at the site of an ulcer. The underlying corneal stroma becomes over-hydrated with tears from the ocular surface.
- **Endothelialitis** Inflammation specifically of the corneal endothelium is uncommon but can occur with infectious canine hepatitis caused by canine adenovirus-1.

3. Appropriate diagnostic tests

- Ocular reflexes
  - ○ Pupillary light reflex – direct and consensual positive OU
  - ○ Dazzle reflex – positive OU
  - ○ Palpebral reflex – positive OU. This reflex is incomplete in the right eye because of the abnormal corneal contour.
- Menace response – positive OU

Pupil size is helpful in providing information about the presence and type of intraocular disease. The pupil is more likely to be dilated in an eye with glaucoma but miotic with anterior uveitis. Even in the presence of corneal opacity, pupil size can be assessed by illuminating the anterior segment from oblique angles in an attempt to detect a tapetal reflection.

- Examination with a focal light source – slit-lamp biomicroscopy reveals that the diffuse opacity is localised to the cornea and that the anterior chamber depth is normal in both eyes. In the right eye, the peripheral corneal vascularisation is superficial, and the pronounced corneal convexity is the result of increased corneal thickness; the multiple areas of lucency are epithelial bullae.

It is helpful to try to assess the level at which corneal vascularisation occurs because this information can help to differentiate intraocular disease from ocular surface disease. Deep corneal vascularisation is generally indicative of intraocular disease, e.g. uveitis, glaucoma or deep corneal pathology. Superficial vascularisation is usually associated with ocular surface disease. Deep corneal blood vessels are usually dark red and do not cross the limbus; they are straight because their path is restricted by the collagen lamellae within the stroma. Superficial vessels are characterised as bright red and branching vessels which may be observed crossing the limbus in the dog but not in the cat.

- Schirmer tear test – 21 mm/min OS. This is not performed OD because of the potentially unstable nature of the cornea which could lead to perforation.

- Fluorescein dye – negative staining OS, multifocal small areas of fluorescein uptake OD. Extensive ulceration would have to be present to account for generalised corneal oedema, and so it is unlikely that the corneal ulceration in the right eye is the cause.
- Tonometry – IOP 18 mmHg OS. Tonometry can only be performed near the limbus OD because of the irregular corneal contour – the IOP readings are variable and considered to be unreliable.

The remainder of the ophthalmic examination reveals no additional abnormalities and a general physical examination is unremarkable.

Diagnosis

Based on the information available, a diagnosis of age-related corneal endothelial degeneration is made.

Treatment

No treatment is indicated in the early stages of this disease when there is only mild corneal oedema, as identified in the left eye of this dog. In more advanced cases, a topical hyperosmotic agent (5% sodium chloride ointment) can be used to reduce the extent of the oedema, although it rarely improves corneal clarity significantly and may cause ocular irritation. Corneal ulcers should be managed with topical broad-spectrum antibiotics in conjunction with systemic analgesic and anti-inflammatory treatment as necessary. Topical atropine is also beneficial to treat associated reflex uveitis if present. Topical lubricants such as a carbomer polymer gel, sodium hyaluronate or a paraffin-based ointment can also be used to improve ocular comfort. Dogs with a persistent bullous keratopathy and recurrent ocular discomfort associated with corneal ulceration should be managed surgically. The ideal surgical technique is a penetrating keratoplasty with fresh corneal tissue. This is the standard technique in humans but is infrequently performed in dogs because of poor availability of donor tissue. The most commonly performed surgical procedure for this condition in the dog is a thermokeratoplasty. Thermokeratoplasty involves the creation of multiple superficial corneal burns using a thermocautery unit to create superficial stromal fibrosis (Fig. 8.1d). The resulting vascular response in the cornea (Fig. 8.1e) ultimately leads to the formation of subepithelial scar tissue which acts as a barrier to the accumulation of fluid within the stroma and prevents the

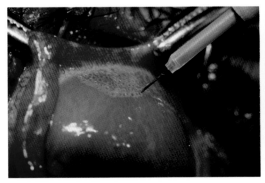

Fig. 8.1d Thermokeratoplasty using a fine diathermy needle.

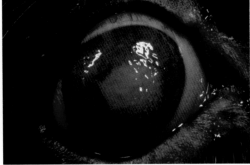

Fig. 8.1e Right eye six weeks postoperatively. Note the multiple points of thermocautery application and the marked corneal vascularisation which progresses in a centripetal direction; the cornea is fluorescein negative.

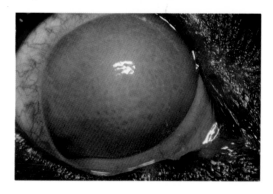

Fig. 8.1f Right eye of a cross-breed dog four months following a thermokeratoplasty performed on the dorsal two-thirds of the cornea.

formation of further bullae. Alternative surgical options that have been described include a superficial keratectomy and/or a thin conjunctival pedicle graft.

Prognosis/Discussion

With age-related corneal endothelial degeneration, corneal oedema is always progressive, albeit at a variable rate between individual dogs and even between the two eyes of the same dog. Once a corneal ulcer develops, it is almost inevitable that future episodes of ulceration will occur. The prognosis for the prevention of corneal ulcer formation following a thermokeratoplasty is good. In a group of 13 dogs with corneal ulcers secondary to endothelial disease (present for a mean of 16.1 weeks), the mean time to healing following thermokeratoplasty was 2.2 ± 1.1 weeks (Michau *et al.*, 2003).

Although a thermokeratoplasty is an effective method of stopping the cyclical corneal pain from corneal ulcers in affected dogs, the prognosis for vision following the procedure is poor. Postoperative corneal scarring can equal or exceed the loss of transparency caused by the corneal oedema (Fig. 8.1f).

References and further reading

Michau TM, Gilger BC, Maggio F, Davidson MG (2003) Use of thermokeratoplasty for treatment of ulcerative keratitis and bullous keratopathy secondary to corneal endothelial disease in dogs: 13 cases (1994–2001). *J Am Vet Med Assoc*, **222**, 607–612.

See Appendix 2.

History

A 5-year-old female neutered English Springer Spaniel is presented with a six-month history of cloudiness in both eyes. The dog has gained weight but is reported to be otherwise clinically well. She has also been routinely vaccinated and receives regular anthelmintic treatment.

Questions

1. Describe the abnormalities and pertinent normal features in Fig. 8.2a.
2. What differential diagnoses should be considered for this presentation?
3. What tests could you perform to make the diagnosis?

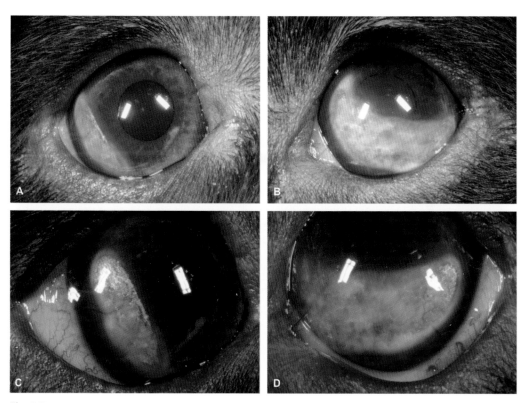

Fig. 8.2a

Answers

1. What the figure shows
Fig. 8.2a Upper images A and B. Both eyes – there is a large focal corneal opacity (OS > OD). The Purkinje images are disrupted where they overlie the corneal opacities but are normal in the areas of clear cornea.

Lower images C and D (magnified view). Both eyes – there is a light grey, scintillating, semi-lunar corneal opacity associated with superficial corneal vascularisation; the opacity is separated from the limbus by clear cornea. The conjunctiva is mildly hyperaemic.

> Corneal transparency is a result of the precise arrangement of collagen fibrils, the relative dehydration of the stroma, and the absence of blood vessels.

2. Differential diagnoses
Based on the appearance of both eyes, the following conditions/explanations for the corneal opacities should be considered:

- **Crystalline corneal opacities**
  - **Lipid keratopathy (corneal lipidosis)** This is a unilateral or bilateral ocular manifestation of systemic disease characterised by peripheral or central grey/white crystalline opacities and a clear perilimbal zone. Bilateral lesions are usually asymmetrical. Corneal vascularisation develops with chronicity. The crystalline opacities are composed of cholesterol, phospholipids and fatty acids. Screening for underlying systemic lipid abnormalities is indicated, e.g. hypothyroidism, pancreatitis, diabetes mellitus, spontaneous hyperlipoproteinaemia and post-prandial plasma lipid elevation.
  - **Corneal dystrophy** This is a primary, bilateral and inherited disorder characterised by central or paracentral grey/white crystalline opacities in the absence of keratitis, vascularisation or systemic disease. Corneal opacities may differ in appearance but are typically bilaterally symmetrical, oval and well-demarcated. They may involve the corneal epithelium, stroma or endothelium and are composed of cholesterol, phospholipids and fatty acids. Affected breeds include the Cavalier King Charles Spaniel, Siberian Husky and Beagle. Diagnostic tests are not usually indicated. Affected dogs should not be used for breeding.
  - **Corneal degeneration** This is usually preceded by keratitis and vascularisation, which, together are the hallmarks of this disease. Corneal lesions are grey/white and crystalline and differ in density; they may be unilateral or bilateral, and poorly defined or well-demarcated. Lesions consist of cholesterol, phospholipids, fatty acids and calcium. The aetiopathogenesis of corneal degeneration is complex and the sequence of events is not always clear. Localised inflammation or injury may cause fibroblasts and keratocytes to produce lipid *in situ*. Alternatively anterior segment inflammation and corneal vascularisation may allow lipid from the systemic circulation to be deposited locally in the cornea. Corneal degeneration can improve with continued vascularisation and phagocytosis – topical corticosteroids should therefore be avoided because of their anti-angiogenic action.
  - **Calcific band keratopathy** This is a specific type of corneal degeneration characterised by a horizontal grey/white crystalline corneal opacity in the interpalpebral fissure. Corneal opacities contain calcium as a result of localised inflammation (dystrophic calcification) or systemic hypercalcaemia (metastatic calcification), e.g. in hyperadrenocorticism.
- **Corneal oedema** Increased hydration of the corneal stroma produces a characteristic dull, blue/grey opacity because of the scattering of light rays (*case 1, this chapter*).

- **Corneal scarring** During stromal healing, new collagen fibres are laid down in a disorganised manner. This causes scattering of light rays which is observed as a corneal opacity. Corneal scars may be focal or generalised, thus reflecting the extent of the initial pathology.

3. Appropriate diagnostic tests
- Ocular reflexes
  - Pupillary light reflex – direct and consensual positive OU
  - Palpebral reflex – positive OU
  - Corneal reflex – positive OU
  - Dazzle reflex – positive OU
- Menace response – positive OU
- Examination with a focal light source – the anterior chamber is normal with respect to depth and transparency OU. Slit-lamp biomicroscopy localises the opacities to the corneal epithelium and anterior stroma and confirms that the corneal vascularisation is superficial.

It is helpful to try to assess the level at which corneal vascularisation occurs because this information can help to differentiate intraocular disease from ocular surface disease. Deep corneal vascularisation is generally indicative of intraocular disease, e.g. uveitis, glaucoma or deep corneal pathology. Superficial vascularisation is usually associated with ocular surface disease. Deep corneal blood vessels are usually dark red and do not cross the limbus; they are straight because their path is restricted by the collagen lamellae within the stroma. Superficial vessels are characterised by being bright red and branching and may be observed crossing the limbus in the dog but not in the cat.

- Schirmer tear test – 18 mm/min OU
- Fluorescein dye
  - Staining – negative OU
  - Tear film break-up time – 18 s OU
- Tonometry – IOP 17 mmHg OU
- Laboratory tests – routine haematology, biochemistry, urine analysis, and screening tests for thyroid and adrenal function reveal abnormalities consistent with hypothyroidism.

A lipid serum profile includes cholesterol and cholesterol esters, triglycerides, total lipids, lipoprotein electrophoresis (high-density and low-density lipoproteins). This profile is not usually performed in the clinical setting as the results do not generally affect case management.

The remainder of the ophthalmic examination reveals no additional abnormalities. A general physical examination indicates an overweight body condition and a slightly dry coat.

Diagnosis
Based on the information available, a diagnosis of lipid keratopathy (corneal lipidosis) associated with hypothyroidism is made.

Treatment
Although not always identified, any underlying disease associated with lipid keratopathy must be treated. Corneal lesions are generally monitored and can be managed both medically and surgically.

Although the efficacy of medical management is unknown, many veterinary ophthalmologists recommend a low-fat diet as well as the topical chelating agent, disodium EDTA (0.40–1.38% in artificial tears) if calcium deposition in the cornea is suspected. Lipid in the cornea, irrespective of the cause, can lead to the development of overlying ulcers which are slow to heal because of the underlying corneal pathology. Surgery in the form of a superficial keratectomy is indicated if the lipid keratopathy is progressive, interferes with vision, causes discomfort and/or delays healing of an ulcer.

In this dog, hypothyroidism is treated with oral thyroxine supplementation and the thyroid function is re-evaluated four to six weeks later. A bilateral keratectomy is performed because the corneal lesion is fairly extensive in both eyes and involves the visual axis in the left eye (Fig. 8.2b). Postoperative management comprises the placement of a soft bandage contact lens to facilitate healing, a topical broad-spectrum antibiotic q8 hours until the surgical site has fully re-epithelialised and systemic NSAID therapy for five days. Histopathology of the cornea reveals multiple clear clefts (Fig. 8.2c, arrow) within the stroma consistent with lipid deposition.

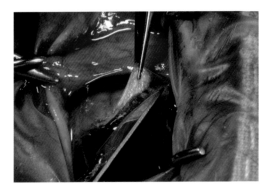

Fig. 8.2b

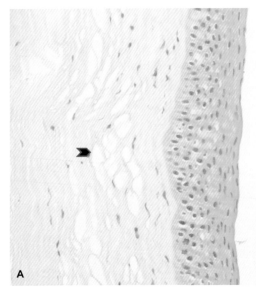

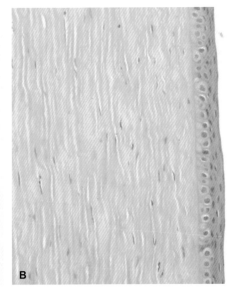

A

B

Fig. 8.2c H & E sections (×200) (A) Multiple clear clefts (arrow) in the corneal stroma consistent with lipid deposition. (B) Normal canine cornea for comparison. Reproduced with permission from EJ Scurrell.

Prognosis

The prognosis for progression of a lipid keratopathy depends on the underlying systemic disease and the treatment elected. If the systemic disease is not identified and/or not well controlled corneal lesions can progress and impair vision. However, if the underlying systemic process is well controlled, the prognosis for the return of corneal transparency following a superficial keratectomy is good.

Discussion

Corneal lipidosis is common in dogs and the clinical appearance alone is often diagnostic. However, it can be challenging to differentiate a lipid keratopathy from a region of corneal degeneration – screening for systemic disease and careful assessment of the presence and degree of corneal vascularisation can be helpful. The diagnosis of corneal dystrophy is usually more straightforward as it is based on a characteristic appearance which is widely described in predisposed breeds.

Further reading

See Appendix 2.

History

A 3-year-old male neutered Persian cat is presented with a two-month history of a black spot on the left eye. The cat has never been in a cattery, and lives indoors in a single cat household. He has been routinely vaccinated, received regular anthelmintic treatment and is otherwise clinically well.

Questions

1. Describe the abnormalities and pertinent normal features in Figs. 8.3a and b.
2. What differential diagnoses should be considered for this presentation?
3. What tests could you perform to make the diagnosis?

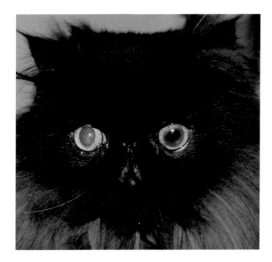

Fig. 8.3a

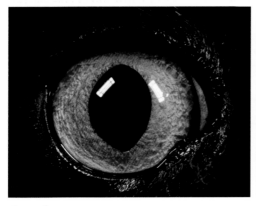
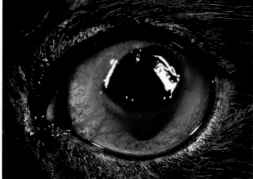

Fig. 8.3b

Answers

1. What the figures show

Fig. 8.3a Both eyes – there is a seromucoid discharge. Left eye – there is an oval black lesion in the axial cornea.

Fig. 8.3b Both eyes – there is mild lower medial entropion. Left eye – a well demarcated, horizontal, oval black corneal lesion is surrounded by oedema and vascularisation. A large vessel extends to this area from the ventromedial region of the limbus. The Purkinje images are disrupted. The anterior chamber is partially obscured by the corneal changes but the iris and anterior chamber appear normal.

2. Differential diagnoses

Given the appearance of the left eye, the following conditions should be considered:

- **Corneal sequestrum (corneal necrosis)** This is a common condition in the cat, particularly in the Persian, and is characterised by brown/black discolouration of the cornea. The affected cornea is degenerate and necrotic. Sequestra can be superficial or deep and can vary considerably in size and in the degree and intensity of associated clinical signs, e.g. pain, discharge, corneal ulceration, and corneal vascularisation.
- **Corneal foreign body** A foreign body such as a flake of paint or a fragment of organic matter can appear as a black corneal opacity. Penetrating and non-penetrating foreign bodies are usually associated with acute ocular discomfort.
- **Corneal pigmentation (melanosis)** Although this is common in the dog, usually as a result of chronic corneal irritation (*case 4, this chapter*), it is not described in the cat.
- **Iris prolapse** Iris tissue can prolapse through a corneal defect following penetrating ocular trauma or perforation of a corneal ulcer. The iris appears as a focal dark grey/black lesion protruding from the corneal surface; there is associated dyscoria. There is often acute pain at the time of the perforation but the eye may become more comfortable within a short time (hours) if the perforation seals with a combination of iris tissue, coagulated aqueous humour, blood and fibrin.
- **Corneal dermoid** This term refers to a congenital choristoma that, in the eye, typically manifests as a focal area of pigmented skin at the temporal limbus, conjunctiva and cornea. Eyelid involvement can occur. A corneal dermoid affecting the central cornea is unusual but has been reported in the dog.
- **Ruptured iris cyst** Uveal cysts usually appear as brown/black spherical structures in the anterior chamber but can create a focal dark corneal opacity following rupture and adherence to the corneal endothelium (*Ch. 9, case 1*).
- **Melanocytic neoplasm** Corneal involvement by a melanocytic neoplasm has only been described in association with the limbus, i.e. limbal melanoma. This benign neoplasm originates from the limbus and appears as a focal black mass. Limbal melanomas can extend locally into adjacent cornea and sclera – therefore involvement of the axial cornea is only observed as a direct extension from the limbus and not as an isolated black lesion.

3. Appropriate diagnostic tests

- Ocular reflexes
  - Pupillary light reflexes – direct and consensual positive OU
  - Dazzle reflex – positive OU
  - Palpebral reflex – positive OU
  - Corneal reflex – positive OU
- Menace response – positive OU

- Examination with a focal light source – slit-lamp biomicroscopy demonstrates that the margins of the black lesion involve the deep corneal stroma and that the corneal vessels are both superficial and deep. It is, however, impossible to reliably determine the exact depth of the central portion of the black lesion.

> It is helpful to try to assess the level at which corneal vascularisation occurs because this information can help to differentiate intraocular disease from ocular surface disease. Deep corneal vascularisation is generally indicative of intraocular disease, e.g. uveitis or glaucoma or deep corneal pathology. Superficial vascularisation is usually associated with ocular surface disease. Deep corneal blood vessels are usually dark red and do not cross the limbus; they are straight because their path is restricted by the collagen lamellae within the stroma. Superficial vessels are characterised by being bright red and branching, and may be observed crossing the limbus in the dog but not in the cat.

- Schirmer tear test – 20 mm/min OD, 28 mm/min OS. This is consistent with increased lacrimation in the left eye, most probably because of the corneal pathology.
- Fluorescein dye
  - Staining – positive staining OS, negative OD. In the left eye, there is an irregular band of fluorescein retention which involves approximately 2 mm of the periphery of the black lesion – this is consistent with a narrow lip of corneal epithelium overlying the edge of the lesion (Fig. 8.3c). Fluorescein dye is also evident within the tear film meniscus along the margins of the upper and lower eyelids which is indicative of a good tear film.
  - Tear film break-up time – 17 s OD. This is not performed OS because the extensive corneal pathology would make the result unreliable.
- Tonometry – IOP 19 mmHg OU
- High-frequency ultrasound biomicroscopy (UBM) – this technique is similar to B-mode ultrasonography but uses higher ultrasound frequencies of between 50 and 100 MHz. Tissue resolution is increased approximately 10-fold compared to a 10 MHz ultrasound probe. This allows discrimination between the different corneal layers. UBM facilitates the planning of surgical management of corneal disease but is not widely available because of cost.

  In this cat, UBM confirms that the corneal lesion involves the deep stromal layers, which correlates with the slit-lamp biomicroscopy findings (Fig. 8.3d).

The remainder of the ophthalmic examination no additional abnormalities and a general physical examination is unremarkable.

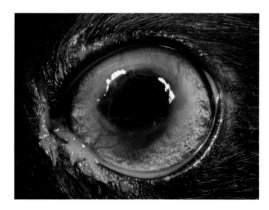

Fig. 8.3c A narrow lip of corneal epithelium overlying the edge of the lesion is delineated by an irregular line of fluorescein retention 2 mm inside the black area. Fluorescein dye is also evident within the tear film meniscus along the margins of the upper and lower eyelids and on the periocular hair.

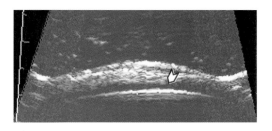

Fig. 8.3d High-frequency ultrasound biomicroscopy scan (cornea). Hyperechoic changes in the deep stroma indicate the depth of the corneal lesion (arrow). Reproduced with permission from E Bentley.

Diagnosis

Based on the information available, a diagnosis of feline corneal sequestrum in the left eye is made.

Treatment

The choice of treatment for a corneal sequestrum depends on several factors, including the degree of corneal involvement and ocular discomfort. The sequestrum begins as a light brown area of discolouration and, if left untreated, progresses to a well-defined black plaque, as is seen in this cat. Over time the sequestrum can be extruded towards the superficial layers of the cornea and eventually slough, as a consequence of corneal healing. Extrusion may take weeks to months and is often associated with ocular discomfort and the risk of corneal perforation. Conservative medical management of a well-tolerated corneal sequestrum includes regular monitoring and topical lubricant and antibiotic therapy. Surgical management in the form of a keratectomy, with or without the placement of a corneal or conjunctival graft, can shorten the course of the disease. It is recommended if there is ocular pain, evidence of secondary bacterial infection and/or the lesion involves the deep layers of the corneal stroma. Grafting of the corneal defect following a keratectomy is often performed to provide tectonic support. Grafting procedures include: conjunctival graft, corneoconjunctival transposition graft, graft using porcine small intestinal submucosa, and a penetrating keratoplasty.

This cat requires a deep keratectomy to completely excise the corneal sequestrum and a corneoconjunctival transposition (CCT) graft to repair the defect (Fig. 8.3e). A CCT graft is a sliding advancement graft which comprises three distinct components: partial thickness peripheral cornea, limbal tissue and adjacent conjunctiva. The CCT graft provides better corneal clarity than a conjunctival graft and is particularly suited to axial corneal lesions (Fig. 8.3e, C). A CCT graft also provides more mechanical support than a conjunctival graft. This is particularly important for a full thickness sequestrum and highlights the importance of trying to establish the depth of the lesion preoperatively. Protocols for preoperative medication differ but include topical broad-spectrum antibiotic and mydriatic/cycloplegic therapy and systemic antibiotics and NSAIDs.

Prognosis

Although the prognosis for a corneal sequestrum is generally good with appropriate case management, recurrence is a well-described feature of the condition. A sequestrum can recur whether or not surgery is performed, although placement of a graft following surgery may help to prevent recurrence. The owner should be cautioned about the risk of development of a sequestrum in the contralateral eye because the disease is often bilateral in pure-breed cats such as the Persian, Himalayan, and Burmese.

Discussion

The exact aetiopathogenesis of corneal sequestrum is unknown but several causes have been described and include: chronic corneal ulceration, keratitis, entropion, trichiasis, and iatrogenic effects, e.g. grid keratotomy. More specifically, suboptimal ocular surface health in brachycephalic

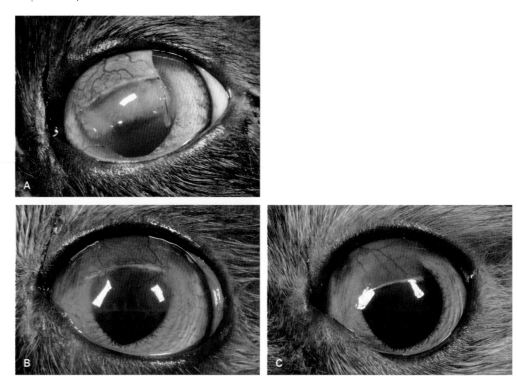

Fig. 8.3e Corneoconjunctival transposition graft in the left eye. (A) 10 days postoperatively. Note the oedema within the corneal component of the graft distal to the limbus. (B) Four weeks postoperatively. The sutures have resorbed, leaving focal opacities, and the corneal oedema has improved. (C) Six months postoperatively. The transposed cornea distal to the limbus is transparent and provides excellent clarity for the axial cornea.

breeds and a genetic component in pure-breed cats have been identified. The association between FHV-1 and the development of a corneal sequestrum has been speculated but remains unclear. FHV-1 is unlikely to be the inciting factor in brachycephalic breeds in which conformational factors are considered to have an important role. The origin and nature of the corneal discolouration is also unclear but suggestions include melanin and porphyrins from the precorneal tear film.

Further reading
See Appendix 2.

History

A 1-year-old male Pug is presented with a recent history of a change in colour of both eyes. The owners have also noticed that the reflection from the eyes in a photograph is different from that for their other Pug. Both dogs have been routinely vaccinated, receive regular anthelmintic treatment and are otherwise clinically well.

Questions

1. Describe the abnormalities and pertinent normal features in Figs. 8.4a and b.
2. What differential diagnoses should be considered for this presentation?
3. What tests could you perform to make the diagnosis?

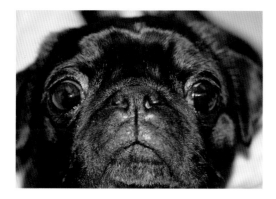

Fig. 8.4a

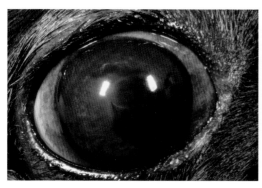
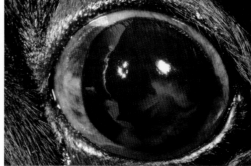

Fig. 8.4b

Answers

1. What the figures show
Fig. 8.4a Both eyes – there is brown pigmentation predominantly of the medial region of the ocular surface. There is no visible tapetal reflection.

Fig. 8.4b Both eyes – the palpebral fissure is oval to round; lower medial entropion is present. The nasal folds are prominent but there is no evidence of trichiasis in either eye. There is increased scleral show (visible sclera around the entire limbus), and conjunctival and corneal pigmentation. The corneal pigmentation is marked (OS > OD) and is mostly restricted to the medial region of the cornea although it covers approximately 70% of the cornea in the left eye. The pigment has a swirling pattern in the axial cornea which is also hazy. The Purkinje images are normal in the right eye but are slightly disrupted in the left eye. The corneal pathology obscures intraocular structures to some extent but the pupil and iris in the right eye appear normal.

2. Differential diagnoses
Given the appearance of both eyes, the clinical diagnosis is bilateral corneal pigmentation (melanosis), for which the following conditions should be considered:

- **Pigmentary keratitis** This term describes bilateral progressive corneal pigmentation and vascularisation which extends from the medial region of the limbus towards the axial cornea. The cause of this syndrome is multifactorial and is related to eyelid conformation in brachycephalic breeds. Predisposing anatomical features include lagophthalmos (caused by a shallow orbit and relative exophthalmos), euryblepharon (or macropalpebral fissure), medial lower entropion, and medial canthal trichiasis. Additional features often include nasal fold trichiasis, distichiasis and keratoconjunctivitis sicca (KCS). All these factors cause chronic ocular surface irritation which leads to the characteristic corneal changes. Not all abnormalities are present in every predisposed breed, e.g. euryblepharon and lagophthalmos are often important factors in the Pug, whereas nasal fold trichiasis is an important cause of ocular surface irritation in the Pekingese. Some authors consider pigmentary keratitis to be a form of corneal dystrophy, particularly if a cause for the corneal irritation cannot be identified.
- **Chronic superficial keratitis (pannus)** An immune-mediated, inflammatory condition of the cornea manifested by bilateral progressive corneal vascularisation and pigmentation which extends from the lateral region of the limbus towards the axial cornea. It is most commonly seen in the German Shepherd Dog, Border Collie and Greyhound but can occur in any breed. Chronic superficial keratitis is commonly associated with plasma cell infiltration of the TEL (*Ch. 3, case 2*).
- **Keratoconjunctivitis sicca (KCS)** Chronic KCS can result in corneal pigmentation in addition to tenacious mucopurulent discharge, conjunctival hyperaemia and thickening, corneal vascularisation and ulceration, reduced vision and discomfort (*Ch. 4, case 4*).

3. Appropriate diagnostic tests
- Ocular reflexes
  - Pupillary light reflex – direct and consensual positive OU
  - Dazzle reflex – positive OU
  - Palpebral reflex – positive but reduced OU
  - Corneal reflex – absent OU
- Menace response – equivocal OS, positive OD

In this dog, these results are consistent with lagophthalmos and reduced corneal sensation in both eyes, and reduced vision in the left eye.

Corneal sensation can be assessed by touching a wisp of cotton wool to the lateral region of the cornea (i.e. away from the visual axis); if a blink response is elicited corneal sensation is said to be present. Corneal sensation can be semi-quantified with a corneal aesthesiometer, e.g. a Cochet-Bonnet or Larson-Millodot aesthesiometer. This instrument consists of a fine filament, which is adjustable in length – the filament is touched to the cornea to elicit a blink. The length of filament required to elicit a blink determines the corneal touch threshold (CTT). CTT is determined in different regions of the cornea. Skull shape influences corneal sensitivity in dogs and cats – the cornea in brachycephalic dogs and cats is less sensitive than in dolichocephalic dog breeds and non-brachycephalic cats.

- Examination with a focal light source – the anterior chamber is normal with respect to depth and transparency in both eyes. Slit-lamp biomicroscopy reveals superficial corneal vascularisation extending from the medial and dorsal regions of the limbus in both eyes. There is a subtle increase in the corneal thickness in the left eye caused by the marked degree of pigment deposition – this accounts for the abnormal Purkinje images noted in Fig. 8.4b.

It is helpful to try to assess the level at which corneal vascularisation occurs because this information can help to differentiate intraocular disease from ocular surface disease. Deep corneal vascularisation is generally indicative of intraocular disease, e.g. uveitis or glaucoma or deep corneal pathology. Superficial vascularisation is usually associated with ocular surface disease. Deep corneal blood vessels are usually dark red and do not cross the limbus; they are straight because their path is restricted by the collagen lamellae within the stroma. Superficial vessels are characterised by being bright red and branching and may be observed crossing the limbus in the dog but not in the cat.

- Ophthalmoscopy – fundic examination is not possible in the left eye because of the extent of the corneal changes. It is performed in the right eye, facilitated by dilating the pupil with tropicamide; no abnormalities are present.
- Schirmer tear test – 15 mm/min OS, 17 mm/min OD. Although these values are within the normal range, tear production may be insufficient for eyes with euryblepharon and lagophthalmos.
- Fluorescein dye
  - Staining – positive 'stippling' of the axial cornea OU. This is consistent with suboptimal ocular surface health but not corneal ulceration in both eyes.
  - Tear film break-up time – 10 s OS, 12 s OD. This is consistent with reduced tear film stability in both eyes.
- Tonometry – IOP 17 mmHg OU

The remainder of the ophthalmic examination reveals no additional abnormalities and a general physical examination is unremarkable. It should be noted that retropulsion of the globe is limited but non-painful in both eyes – this is a common finding in brachycephalic breeds because of their shallow orbits.

Diagnosis
Based on the information available, a diagnosis of pigmentary keratitis is made in both eyes, primarily because of the brachycephalic conformation.

Treatment

The treatment of pigmentary keratitis depends on the underlying cause and the severity of the corneal changes. In dogs with mild conformational abnormalities and early corneal changes, it may be sufficient to treat with topical lubricant therapy, e.g. a paraffin-based ophthalmic ointment, and to monitor for disease progression. More specifically, diagrams and/or photodocumentation will help to identify early or progressive changes. Surgical management is recommended in young dogs with marked conformational abnormalities and secondary corneal disease or if there is evidence of progressive corneal disease which could impair vision. A medial canthoplasty addresses the medial canthal abnormalities (entropion, trichiasis) and will reduce lagophthalmos whereas a lateral canthoplasty will only improve lagophthalmos. Simultaneous medial and lateral canthoplasties may be considered in eyes with extreme euryblepharon. Several techniques are described and the choice is based on the experience and preference of the surgeon. The lower nasolacrimal punctal openings should theoretically be preserved, regardless of procedure chosen, but this limits by how much the palpebral length can be shortened. However, some ophthalmologists sacrifice the punctal openings to maximise retention of the tear film, which is considered to be beneficial to ocular surface health.

Surgery is elected in this dog because of the extent of the corneal pigmentation and the young age. A bilateral medial canthoplasty is performed (Fig. 8.4c). Note the change in size and shape of the palpebral fissure in both eyes from the preoperative stage to the postoperative stage – the large round aperture (Figs. 8.4a and b) becomes smaller and more almond-shaped with no exposed sclera (Fig. 8.4c). Absorbable skin sutures, e.g. 6/0 polyglactin, are ideal for eyelid surgery because removal

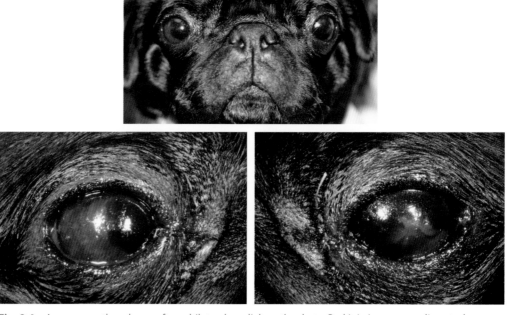

Fig. 8.4c Appearance three hours after a bilateral medial canthoplasty. Purkinje images are disrupted because of topical administration of an antibiotic ointment.

of sutures can be difficult in conscious animals. Postoperative medication comprises topical and systemic broad-spectrum antibiotic and NSAID therapy for seven to ten days. Once the skin wounds have sufficiently healed (usually within two to three weeks), topical anti-inflammatory medication can help to decrease corneal vascularisation and pigmentation, e.g. corticosteroids, cyclosporine, tacrolimus. Brachycephalic breeds are predisposed to corneal ulceration and topical corticosteroid therapy should be used with caution. Although a keratectomy to remove the corneal pigment can be considered (following correction of the conformational abnormalities), it is rarely performed. The procedure is not without risk as corneal healing tends to be delayed in these dogs.

Prognosis
The aim of surgery is not only to halt the progression of the corneal pigmentation but also to reduce the extent and density of the existing pigment to improve corneal clarity. The prognosis is good with early and accurate diagnosis and prompt surgical management. However many dogs do not present until the corneal changes are so advanced that they are visually impaired. Although medical and surgical treatment can help dogs with advanced disease, the beneficial effects are more likely to be seen in the overall ocular surface health rather than in significantly improved vision.

Discussion
Corneal pigmentation is a result of the migration of melanocytic cells from the limbal and per-ilimbal tissues. Melanin pigment is deposited in the basal epithelial cells and the superficial stroma, and is found in macrophages and fibroblasts. Corneal pigmentation is a common feature of chronic ocular surface disease in the dog, but does not occur in the cat (*case 3, this chapter*); the reason for this is unknown. This case of pigmentary keratitis describes the management of chronic ocular surface disease with the emphasis on surgical treatment, but the importance of ocular surface lubrication with artificial tear preparations for promoting corneal healing should also be emphasised.

This case highlights how brachycephalic conformation (macropalpebral fissure, lagophthalmos, exophthalmos) has a profound influence on ocular surface health. This influence may only become apparent when the ocular surface is challenged. For example, a simple corneal ulcer can become complicated within a short time in a brachycephalic dog. From the outset the clinician has the ability to prescribe treatment that can either promote or delay corneal healing, and an inappropriate choice of treatment can cause the ulcer to deteriorate rapidly. Topical ocular preparations have harmful as well as beneficial effects on healing and ocular surface health. The choice of drug is particularly pertinent when treating brachycephalic breeds with suboptimal ocular surface health. All antibiotics have epitheliotoxic effects, but some, e.g. gentamicin and ciprofloxacin, profoundly limit the ability of the cornea to heal and should be avoided in eyes with poor epithelial healing, particularly when alternative antibiotics, e.g. chloramphenicol, are just as likely to be effective. Topical atropine is used in the management of corneal ulcers for its cycloplegic and mydriatic properties. However, atropine reduces tear production, which in turn can delay corneal healing. This is especially relevant in brachycephalic breeds, where tear production is often marginal and ocular surface health is com-promised. In these breeds atropine should be used at the minimum frequency required to maintain cycloplegia.

Further reading
See Appendix 2.

CHAPTER 9

Abnormalities of the Iris

Introduction

The iris forms the anterior part of the uveal tract, which is the highly vascular, usually pigmented, layer of the eye. The function of the iris is to control the amount of light entering the posterior aspect of the eye through a central pupil. The iris is closely associated with the lens and consequently has a curvature similar to the anterior surface of the lens; if the lens is displaced this can result in a change in position of the iris. In general, the pathology of the uvea reflects its purpose as the primary vascular source of the globe and the role it plays in the inflammatory process. With the exception of inflammation and neoplasia, abnormalities of the iris are relatively uncommon, but are readily observed because of the anterior location of the iris.

Small Animal Ophthalmology: What's Your Diagnosis? First Edition. Heidi Featherstone, Elaine Holt.
© 2011 by Heidi Featherstone and Elaine Holt. Published 2011 by Blackwell Publishing Ltd.

History

A 9-year-old female neutered Staffordshire Bull Terrier is presented with a six-month history of progressive visual impairment. The dog has received routine vaccinations and anthelmintic treatment and is otherwise clinically well.

Questions

1. Describe the abnormalities and pertinent normal features in Figs. 9.1a and b.
2. What differential diagnoses should be considered for this presentation?
3. What tests could you perform to make the diagnosis?

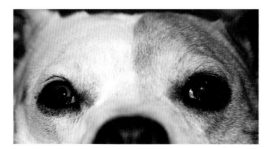

Fig. 9.1a

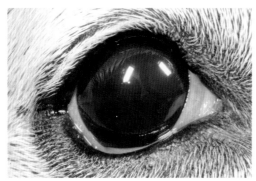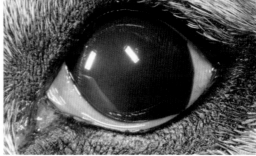

Fig. 9.1b

Answers

1. What the figures show
Fig. 9.1a Both eyes – the tapetal reflection is absent in the left eye and is obscured by a dark brown area which overlies the ventrolateral region of the pupil in the right eye. The Purkinje images are normal.

Fig. 9.1b Left eye – there is subtle corneal oedema. Right eye – there are multiple dark brown spherical structures in the anterior chamber.

2. What differential diagnoses should be considered?
Based on the appearance of the right eye and given the consideration that the condition may be bilateral, the following conditions should be considered:

- **Uveal cyst(s)** Cysts arise from the accumulation of fluid between the bilayered epithelium of the posterior iris or ciliary body. Cysts are common in the dog and may be congenital or acquired following trauma or uveitis. They can be unilateral or bilateral, single or multiple, of different sizes, and are usually brown or black. Cysts are often free-floating within the anterior chamber but can also remain attached to the posterior iris or ciliary body where they can only be observed following mydriasis. Collapsed cysts are common and result in focal areas of pigment on the corneal endothelium or anterior lens capsule. Uveal cysts are common in the Golden Retriever, Labrador Retriever and Boston Terrier, but can occur in any breed of dog. It is important to differentiate a uveal cyst from a melanocytic neoplasm; cysts are generally easily identified by their clinical appearance and with the aid of transillumination (Diagram 9.1).

- **Melanocytic neoplasm** This is the most common primary intraocular neoplasm in the dog. Intraocular melanocytic neoplasia in the dog is divided into two groups: benign melanocytoma and malignant melanoma. Intraocular melanocytic neoplasia is most common in middle-aged dogs with a mean age of 9 years, although an age range of two months to 17 years has been

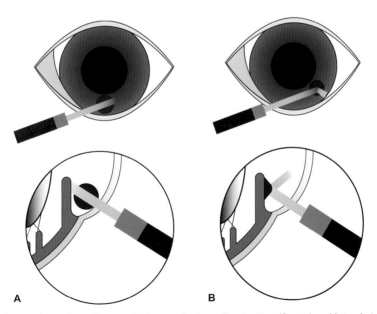

Diagram 9.1 Comparison of uveal cyst and iris mass by transillumination (frontal and lateral view). (A) Light beam passes through the cyst. (B) Light beam is deflected from the surface of a solid iris mass. Illustration by S Scurrell.

reported. Melanocytomas are more common than malignant melanomas; both forms arise most frequently in the anterior uvea (iris and ciliary body), and are usually nodular rather than diffuse, in contrast to the cat (*case 3, this chapter*). The clinical appearance of a melanocytic neoplasm can vary from a focal colour change within the iris to a single mass protruding through the pupil; the mass can be large enough to cause dyscoria, uveitis and secondary glaucoma. Owners may observe a colour change or mass effect in the eye or might only notice ocular discomfort, redness or impaired vision caused by the secondary uveitis or glaucoma. Choroidal melanocytomas and malignant melanomas do occur but are less common. Because of their location in the posterior segment, diagnosis is often late, by which time the tumours have reached a large size and may be accompanied by retinal detachment.

- **Metastatic neoplasia** Neoplasms can metastasise haematogenously to the eye from local or distant sites or can invade the eye by direct local extension. Bilateral ocular involvement is characteristic of metastatic neoplasia, in contrast to the unilateral occurrence of primary ocular neoplasia. The uveal tract is a predilection site for haematogenous spread and metastatic neoplasia is consequently associated with uveitis and secondary glaucoma. Gross observation of metastatic neoplasia is often not possible because a mass lesion does not necessarily occur. Lymphoma is the most common secondary neoplasm in the eye; other examples include mammary gland adenocarcinoma, transitional cell carcinoma, haemangiosarcoma and osteosarcoma.
- **Chronic anterior uveitis** Chronic uveitis often causes darkening of the iris because of diffuse iridal hyperpigmentation (as a result of pigment proliferation and migration) and hyperaemia, and is most obvious in lightly pigmented irides. Other signs of chronic uveitis are usually present and include corneal oedema, keratic precipitates, rubeosis iridis, posterior synechiae, iris rests, secondary cataract, and hypotony.

3. Appropriate diagnostic tests

- Ocular reflexes
  - Pupillary light reflex – the left pupil is not visible. Consensual positive OS (left to right eye), direct positive OD.
  - Dazzle reflex – positive OU
- Vision assessment
  - Menace response – equivocal OS, positive OD
  - Visual placing and tracking reflexes – positive OU
  - Obstacle course – the dog can navigate around large objects in both photopic and scotopic conditions.

  In this dog, these results suggest reduced vision in the left eye.

- Examination with a focal light source – there are multiple dark brown spherical structures in the anterior chamber of the left eye. Some of the spherical structures can be transilluminated (Diagram 9.1). Slit-lamp biomicroscopy reveals a subtle increase in corneal thickness in the left eye because of corneal oedema, an increase in the depth of the anterior chamber, and a dark brown iris of apparently normal thickness in both eyes.
- Schirmer tear test – 17 mm/min OU
- Tonometry – IOP 28 mmHg OU
- Gonioscopy – observation of the filtration angle is prevented by the corneal oedema in the left eye. The multiple brown spherical structures in the anterior chamber of both eyes also prohibit gonioscopy.
- B-mode ultrasound – this confirms the presence of multiple, spherical fluid-filled structures within the anterior chamber of both eyes (Fig. 9.1c).

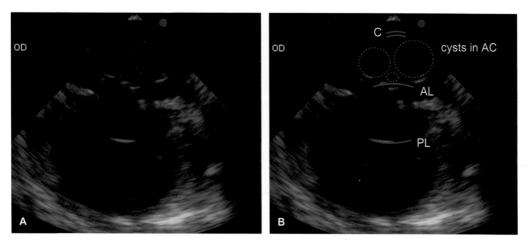

Fig. 9.1c (A) B-mode ultrasound image of the right eye. (B). Annotated image showing multiple fluid-filled structures (uveal cysts) with a hyperechoic wall in the anterior chamber. AC, anterior chamber; C, cornea; AL, anterior surface of the lens; PL, posterior surface of the lens.

The remainder of the ophthalmic examination reveals no additional abnormalities and a general physical examination is unremarkable.

Diagnosis
Based on the information available, a diagnosis of uveal cysts is made in both eyes.

Treatment
Most uveal cysts are clinically insignificant but possible adverse effects include visual impairment and damage to the corneal endothelium (because of direct contact). Interference with aqueous humour drainage, either by physical obstruction of the entrance to the filtration angle or anterior displacement of the iris resulting in angle closure, can also occur. Treatment options for uveal cysts include aspiration with a needle, laser ablation and surgical removal with combined aspiration and irrigation. Aspiration (by a needle inserted into the anterior chamber from the limbus, *Ch. 7, case 2, Fig. 7.2c*) is appropriate for a large, single, and accessible cyst. Laser ablation can be performed under sedation or general anaesthesia with an Nd:YAG or diode laser. Darkly pigmented cysts are more amenable to laser therapy as the laser energy is absorbed by melanin. Although laser ablation is reported to be an effective and safe technique, in the authors' experience it can cause corneal damage (oedema, scarring) in eyes with a high number of cysts.

Removal of the cysts is indicated in this dog because of the history of visual impairment, the evidence of endothelial damage (corneal oedema) in the left eye and the slightly elevated intraocular pressure in both eyes. Surgical removal by combined aspiration and irrigation is chosen because of the unusually high number of cysts in both eyes. Surgery is performed with the aid of an operating microscope – a clear corneal incision results in the immediate escape of aqueous humour and several cysts; the remaining cysts are removed by careful aspiration facilitated by the use of viscoelastic (Fig. 9.1d, A). Several cyst wall remnants become adhered to the corneal endothelium in both eyes and are left *in situ* because attempted removal would be likely to damage the endothelial cells (Fig. 9.1d, B). Postoperative medication comprises topical atropine and 1% prednisolone acetate as well as systemic NSAID therapy for two weeks. The dog is monitored regularly for further cyst development – both eyes remain visual and normotensive one year after surgery (Fig. 9.1e).

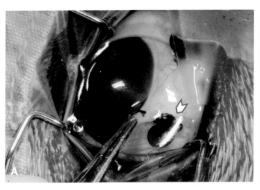
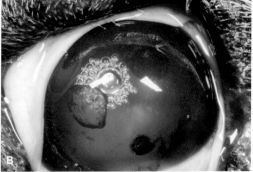

Fig. 9.1d (A) Cysts and aqueous humour exit the anterior chamber following the corneal incision (left eye). (B) Relatively clear anterior chamber and dilated pupil at the end of surgery (left eye). Three cyst wall remnants are adherent to the corneal endothelium. There are air bubbles in the aqueous humour and viscoelastic, some of which is retained following corneal closure.

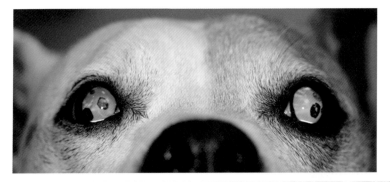

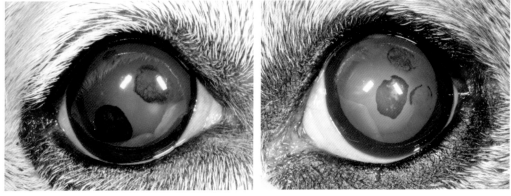

Fig. 9.1e Appearance one year after surgery (pupils have been dilated with tropicamide) – the visual axes are clear apart from several cyst wall remnants adherent to the corneal endothelium.

Prognosis

The prognosis for a visual, comfortable, and normotensive eye following cyst removal is excellent, regardless of the technique used. A retrospective study on the use of a semiconductor diode laser for the removal of uveal cysts in dogs, cats and horses, described a success rate of 100% (Gemensky-Metzler *et al.*, 2004). The adherence of cyst wall remnants to the corneal endothelium can lead to

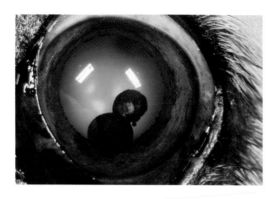

Fig. 9.1f Two uveal cysts in the anterior chamber of a young adult Labrador.

chronic focal corneal oedema and subsequent corneal ulceration. The development of further cysts is a possible sequela, especially in eyes with numerous cysts.

Discussion

This dog is unusual with respect to the high number of cysts affecting both eyes – the more typical presentation is a single cyst or a low number of cysts in one eye (Fig. 9.1f).

Although uveal cysts are generally benign, there are two different breed-related syndromes that demonstrate an association between cysts and glaucoma. Great Danes can be affected with multiple cysts in the posterior chamber that cause anterior displacement of the iris and secondary glaucoma. In Golden Retrievers, a syndrome referred to as pigmentary uveitis is characterised by multiple iridociliary cysts and concurrent uveitis and glaucoma. The cysts are not always visible on routine ophthalmic examination and may only be identified on histopathology. The exact causal relationship between the cysts and uveitis is unknown.

References and further reading

Gemensky-Metzler AJ, Wilkie DA, Cook CS (2004) The use of semiconductor diode laser for deflation and coagulation of anterior uveal cysts in dogs, cats, horses: a report of 20 cases. *Vet Ophthalmol*, **7** (5), 360–368.

See Appendix 2.

History

A 4-year-old female neutered Siberian Husky is presented with a three-month history of a dark spot in the right eye. The dog has received routine vaccinations and anthelmintic treatment and is otherwise clinically well.

Questions

1. Describe the abnormalities and pertinent normal features in Figs. 9.2a and b.
2. What differential diagnoses should be considered for this presentation?
3. What tests could you perform to make the diagnosis?

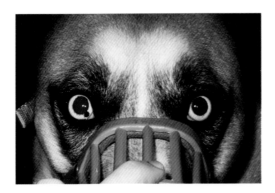

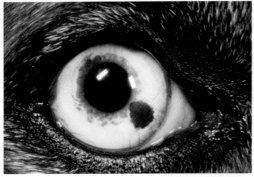
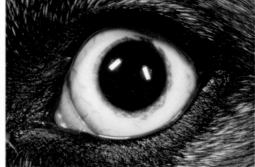

Fig. 9.2a

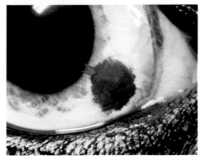

Fig. 9.2b

Answers

1. What the figures show

Figs. 9.2a and b The left eye is normal. There is a relative anisocoria (OD < OS) caused by ambient lighting. Right eye – there is a focal, well-demarcated, dark brown circular lesion in the ventrolateral quadrant of the iris. The lesion does not appear to extend to the pupil margin or the peripheral iris. The limbus is partially pigmented (visible in the dorsomedial region of the eye) which is a common, normal variation in the dog. The Purkinje images are normal.

2. Differential diagnoses

Given the appearance of the right eye, the following conditions should be considered:

- **Melanocytic neoplasm** This is the most common primary intraocular neoplasm in the dog. Intraocular melanocytic neoplasia in the dog is divided into two groups – benign melanocytoma and malignant melanoma. Intraocular melanocytic neoplasms are most common in middle-aged dogs (a mean age of 9 years, age range of two months to 17 years has been reported). Melanocytomas are more common than malignant melanomas; both forms arise most frequently in the anterior uvea (iris and ciliary body), and are usually nodular rather than diffuse, in contrast to the cat (*case 3, this chapter*). The clinical appearance of a melanocytic neoplasm can vary from a focal colour change within the iris to a single mass protruding through the pupil; the mass can be large enough to cause dyscoria, uveitis and secondary glaucoma. Owners may observe a colour change or mass effect in the eye or might only notice ocular discomfort, redness or impaired vision caused by the secondary uveitis or glaucoma. Choroidal melanocytomas and malignant melanomas do occur but are less common. Because of their location in the posterior segment, diagnosis is often late, by which time the tumours have become large and they may be accompanied by retinal detachment. The risk of metastatic disease for melanocytic neoplasms will be described later.

- **Iridociliary epithelial tumour (adenoma, adenocarcinoma)** This is the second most common primary intraocular tumour in the dog. This tumour arises from the pigmented or non-pigmented cells of the iris or the ciliary body and can appear as a mass within the pupil and/or can involve the iris. These tumours can be difficult to distinguish from melanocytic neoplasia by clinical appearance alone. Even in the case of a locally invasive iridociliary adenocarcinoma, the risk of metastatic disease is low.

- **Miscellaneous primary neoplasia** Other primary intraocular tumours are uncommon in the dog. They include medulloepithelioma, spindle cell tumour, haemangioma, haemangiosarcoma, leiyomyoma, leiyomyosarcoma, and osteosarcoma. A medulloepithelioma is a congenital tumour which arises from the neuroectoderm layer of the optic cup. In the dog the tumour most commonly originates in the ciliary body and appears as a grey/white mass within the pupil or as a mass extending through the iris. Spindle cell tumours of the uveal tract are thought to originate from peripheral nerve tissue in blue irides in breeds such as the Siberian Husky; the tumour appears as a nodular non-pigmented mass. Although locally infiltrative, metastatic disease has not been reported.

- **Metastatic neoplasia** Neoplasia can metastasise haematogenously to the eye from local or distant sites or can invade the eye by direct local extension. Bilateral ocular involvement is characteristic of metastatic neoplasia, in contrast to the unilateral occurrence of primary ocular neoplasia. The uveal tract is a predilection site for haematogenous spread and metastatic neoplasia is consequently associated with uveitis and secondary glaucoma. Gross observation of metastatic neoplasia is often not possible because a mass lesion does not necessarily occur. Lymphoma is the most common secondary neoplasm in the eye; other examples include mammary gland adenocarcinoma, transitional cell carcinoma, haemangiosarcoma and osteosarcoma.

- **Benign iris hyperpigmentation or iris freckle (benign melanosis, pigment cell clusters)** An iris freckle appears as a well-circumscribed, non-elevated area of iridal hyperpigmentation as a result of increased melanin within the melanocytes without an increase in melanocyte number; lesions may be single or multiple. Iris freckles usually develop with increasing age and are therefore most commonly seen as a bilateral condition in geriatric dogs.
- **Iris nevus** A nevus appears as a well-circumscribed, slightly elevated area of hyperpigmentation of the iris as a result of melanocyte proliferation. Nevi are usually non-progressive but may undergo malignant transformation. Lesions tend to be single and often occur in young dogs.
- **Uveal cyst(s)** Cysts arise from the accumulation of fluid between the bilayered epithelium of the posterior iris or ciliary body. Cysts are common in the dog and may be congenital or acquired, following trauma or uveitis. They can be unilateral or bilateral, single or multiple, of different sizes, and are usually brown or black (*case 1, this chapter*). Cysts are often free-floating within the anterior chamber but can also remain attached to the posterior iris or ciliary body where they can only be observed following mydriasis. Collapsed cysts are common and result in focal areas of pigment on the corneal endothelium or anterior lens capsule. Uveal cysts are common in the Golden Retriever, Labrador Retriever and Boston Terrier, but can occur in any breed of dog. It is important to differentiate a uveal cyst from a melanocytic neoplasm; cysts are generally easily identified by their clinical appearance and with the aid of transillumination (*case 1, this chapter, Diagram 9.1*).
- **Melanocytosis (ocular melanosis, pigmentary glaucoma, abnormal ocular pigment deposition and glaucoma)** This term refers to a syndrome characterised by the proliferation of pigmented cells (melanocytes and melanophages) throughout the uvea. It has been described primarily in the Cairn Terrier and also in the Golden Retriever, Labrador Retriever and Boxer. It is invariably a bilateral condition in the Cairn Terrier but can be unilateral or bilateral in other breeds. Hyperpigmentation involves the iris, the ciliary body, choroid and filtration angle. The iris typically appears diffusely thickened and patches of pigment develop in the episclera posterior to the limbus. Secondary glaucoma is common as a result of pigmented cells obstructing the ciliary cleft and trabecular meshwork. In the Cairn Terrier, ultrastructural evaluation of the pigmented cells has confirmed that they are predominantly melanocytes and not just melanophages (macrophages containing phagocytosed melanin pigment) (Petersen-Jones *et al.*, 2008).

3. Appropriate diagnostic tests
- Ocular reflexes
  - Pupillary light reflex – direct and consensual positive OU
  - Dazzle reflex – positive OU
- Menace response – positive OU
- Examination with a focal light source – there is no evidence of iris thickening associated with the area of hyperpigmentation in the right eye. Slit-lamp biomicroscopy reveals a subtle change in the surface texture of the pigmented area compared with that of the adjacent iris.
- Schirmer tear test – 17 mm/min OU
- Tonometry – IOP 18 mmHg OU

The remainder of the ophthalmic examination reveals no additional abnormalities and a general physical examination is unremarkable.

Diagnosis
Based on the information available, a presumptive diagnosis of iris melanocytoma in the right eye is made.

Treatment

Treatment for an intraocular melanocytic neoplasm in the dog depends on several factors including the extent of the lesion, the overall health of the eye and the dog, the presence of metastatic disease, financial considerations, available equipment and the skills of the surgeon. Careful monitoring for disease progression is appropriate for small lesions. Treatment options for more advanced disease include diode laser photocoagulation, local excision by sector iridectomy, enucleation and exenteration. For photocoagulation, the lesion should be confined to the iris and have no concurrent complicating factors such as uveitis or glaucoma. For local excision by sector iridectomy, the optimal lesion is one that is well-defined, confined to the iris and located axial to the major arterial circle in the peripheral iris. Enucleation is generally reserved for a blind and painful eye in a dog with no evidence of metastatic disease. Exenteration should be performed when there is evidence of extraocular extension of the neoplasm into the orbit.

In this dog, both photocoagulation and sector iridectomy are considered – the former is elected because of the risks of haemorrhage and the potential for incomplete excision with sector iridectomy.

Topical 1% pilocarpine is administered preoperatively to induce miosis in order to provide good exposure of the maximal surface area of the lesion (Fig. 9.2c). The dog is placed under general anaesthesia – a diode laser unit in combination with a laser indirect ophthalmoscope and a 20D condensing lens is used to treat the lesion. Laser energy is directed at the lesion until there is no further reduction in size. Minor dyscoria is noted at the end of the procedure, a common and acceptable finding following laser treatment (Fig. 9.2d). Postoperative treatment comprises topical 1% prednisolone acetate and 0.5% atropine for 10 days. Atropine is used to minimise the risk of the formation of posterior synechiae and pain associated with miosis (the latter as a result of the preoperative topical pilocarpine and the postoperative uveitis). An ocular examination for signs of recurrence is performed after three months, six months and one year, and annually thereafter. There are no signs of recurrence in this dog two years after the laser therapy.

Prognosis

The prognosis for vision and a complete cure for an ocular melanocytoma in the dog appears to be good following diode laser photocoagulation. However, this information is based on only one study

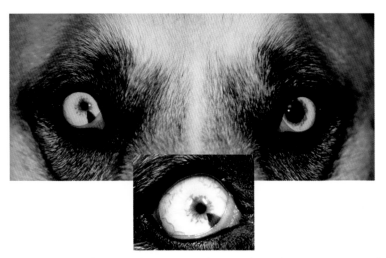

Fig. 9.2c Miosis in the right eye following the topical application of 1% pilocarpine to expose the maximum surface area of the lesion.

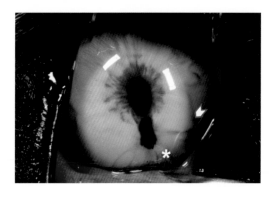

Fig. 9.2d Appearance of the iris following diode laser photocoagulation. Note the overall reduction in size of the lesion, mild dyscoria, hyperaemia of the iris vessels (asterix) and the proximity of the major arterial circle (arrow) to the lesion.

in the veterinary literature (Cook & Wilkie, 1999). In that study repeat laser therapy was required in five of the 23 dogs but there was no clinical evidence of disease recurrence following the last treatment in all dogs; follow-up ranged from 6 months to 4.5 years. Minor complications of photocoagulation include dyscoria (as occurred in this dog), iris hyperpigmentation and corneal oedema. Major complications include cataract and glaucoma. The prognosis for survival is excellent for dogs that undergo enucleation and have a clinical diagnosis of melanocytoma confirmed with ocular histopathology. The prognosis for recurrence of the disease and for the eye itself following sector iridectomy is fair to guarded, as incomplete excision and complications associated with intraocular haemorrhage can occur.

Discussion

The majority of melanocytic uveal tumours are benign in the dog. Malignant melanomas are less common and carry a low potential for metastasis (4–10%). This, together with the unproven efficacy of enucleation at preventing metastasis from a malignant melanoma, makes it difficult to recommend removal of a comfortable, visual, and non-inflamed eye and it is appropriate to consider other surgical procedures. Although fine needle aspiration of a suspected melanocytic neoplasm is ideal, obtaining a representative cellular sample of a pigmented iris lesion is challenging and generally unrewarding, and it is therefore not routinely performed in veterinary medicine. Generally, if the clinical appearance and behaviour of the lesion is characteristic for a benign process, as in this dog, the risks associated with an invasive biopsy procedure outweigh the possible diagnostic value. This is particularly true for isolated iris lesions without complicating factors such as uveitis and glaucoma. In contrast to the situation in the dog, diffuse iris melanoma in the cat is associated with a greater risk of metastatic disease and for this reason pigmented iris lesions in the cat are not usually managed with laser photocoagulation (*case 3, this chapter*).

References and further reading

Cook CS & Wilkie DA (1999) Treatment of presumed iris melanoma in dogs by diode laser photocoagulation: 23 cases. *Vet Ophthalmol*, **2**, 217–225.

Giuliano EA, Chappell R, Fischer B, Dubielzig RR (1999) A matched observational study of canine survival with primary intraocular melanocytic neoplasia. *Vet Ophthalmol*, **2**, 185–190.

Petersen-Jones SM, Mentzer AL, Dubielzig RR, Render JA, Steficek BA, Kiupel M (2008) Ocular melanosis in the Cairn Terrier: histopathological description of the condition, and immunohistochemical and ultrastructural characterisation of the characteristic pigment-laden cells. *Vet Ophthalmol*, **11** (4), 260–268.

See Appendix 2.

History

A 12-year-old female neutered domestic shorthaired cat is presented with a six-month history of a colour change in the right eye. The cat lives with another aged cat and they have both received routine vaccinations and regular anthelmintic treatment up until the last year; they are indoor/outdoor cats.

Questions

1. Describe the abnormalities and pertinent normal features in Fig. 9.3a.
2. What differential diagnoses should be considered for this presentation?
3. What tests could you perform to make the diagnosis?

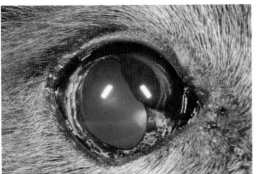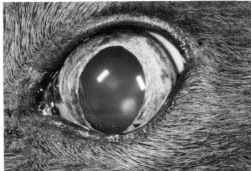

Fig. 9.3a

Answers

1. What the figure shows

Fig. 9.3a Both eyes – the pupils appear opalescent because of age-related nuclear sclerosis. The Purkinje images are normal. Left eye – there is multifocal hyperpigmentation of the iris. Right eye – there is multifocal hyperpigmentation of the iris and a large, well-defined dark brown mass in the dorsomedial iris which extends from 12 to 3 o'clock and results in dyscoria.

2. Differential diagnoses

Given the appearance of both eyes, the following conditions should be considered:

- **Diffuse iris melanoma (DIM)** This is the most common primary intraocular neoplasm in the cat, and typically presents as a unilateral progressive hyperpigmentation of the iris over months to years. Hyperpigmentation can occur as a single area on the anterior surface of the iris or as multiple areas which become confluent with time. The earliest clinical sign of DIM is iridal hyperpigmentation, followed by a subtle velveteen change in the iris surface texture, iris thickening, dyscoria, reduced pupil mobility, pigment within the aqueous humour, and clinical signs of anterior uveitis; the presence of secondary glaucoma is consistent with advanced disease.
- **Benign iridal melanosis** This term refers to a proliferation of melanocytes which is restricted to the anterior surface of the iris. Diffuse iridal hyperpigmentation occurs when multiple lesions coalesce, and can be difficult to clinically differentiate from DIM. Benign melanosis usually develops with increasing age and is therefore most commonly seen as a bilateral condition in geriatric cats.
- **Chronic anterior uveitis** Chronic uveitis often causes darkening of the iris because of diffuse iridal hyperpigmentation (as a result of pigment proliferation and migration) and is most obvious in lightly pigmented irides. Other signs of chronic uveitis are usually present and include corneal oedema, keratic precipitates, rubeosis iridis, posterior synechiae, iris rests, secondary cataract, and hypotony.
- **Uveal cyst(s)** In contrast to the dog, this is an uncommon lesion in the cat. Cysts result from an accumulation of fluid within the bilayered epithelium of the posterior iris or ciliary body. In the cat, uveal cysts are usually dark brown/black, and remain attached to the pupillary margin or the posterior surface of the iris. Multiple cysts are more common than single cysts. It is important to differentiate a uveal cyst from a uveal neoplasm such as a melanoma – cysts are generally easily identified by their clinical appearance and with the aid of transillumination (*case 1, this chapter, Diagram 9.1*).
- **Feline post-traumatic ocular sarcoma** This is an uncommon but highly malignant neoplasm, usually associated with a previous history of ocular trauma and lens injury. The clinical presentation is unilateral and can include signs of chronic uveitis, glaucoma, intraocular haemorrhage and a white/pink mass in the posterior segment of the eye.
- **Iridociliary epithelial tumour (adenoma, adenocarcinoma)** These tumours arise from pigmented or non-pigmented cells of the iris or ciliary body and typically appear as a non-pigmented mass within the pupil or at the iris root. They are uncommon in cats.
- **Lymphoma** Lymphoma is the most common metastatic intraocular tumour in the cat. It can appear as anterior uveitis, or a pink/white mass in the anterior chamber, or both. In contrast to the dog, the majority of cats present with a nodular iris mass rather than with diffuse iris thickening. Although ocular lymphoma in the cat is generally considered to be a manifestation of multisystemic disease, primary ocular lymphoma may occur. Aqueous humour cytology is frequently diagnostic as the tumour exfoliates cells readily.
- **Metastatic neoplasia** Neoplasia can metastasise haematogenously to the eye from local or distant sites or can invade the eye by direct local extension. Bilateral ocular involvement is char-

acteristic of metastatic neoplasia, in contrast to the unilateral occurrence of primary ocular neoplasia. The uveal tract is a predilection site for haematogenous spread and metastatic neoplasia is consequently associated with uveitis and secondary glaucoma. Gross observation of metastatic neoplasia is often not possible because there may not be a mass lesion. Lymphoma is the most common secondary neoplasm in the eye; other examples include mammary gland adenocarcinoma, transitional cell carcinoma, haemangiosarcoma and osteosarcoma.

3. Appropriate diagnostic tests
- Ocular reflexes
  - Pupillary light reflex – direct and consensual positive OU. There is reduced mobility of the right pupil.
  - Dazzle reflex – positive OU
- Menace response – positive OU
- Examination with a focal light source – this reveals an iridal mass which obliterates the anterior chamber in the dorsomedial quadrant of the right eye and almost contacts the adjacent corneal endothelium. Slit-lamp biomicroscopy reveals that the hyperpigmented areas have a velveteen appearance and are thickened. This is in contrast to the hyperpigmented areas in the left eye which appear normal with respect to surface texture and thickness.
- Schirmer tear test – 10 mm/min OU
- Fluorescein dye – negative staining OU
- Tonometry – IOP 17 mmHg OS, 20 mmHg OD
- Gonioscopy – normal filtration angle OS, abnormal filtration angle OD. The filtration angle in the right eye is infiltrated by the iris mass in the dorsomedial quadrant.

> Visualisation of the filtration angle can often be performed without the use of a goniolens in the cat because of a deep anterior chamber in this species.

The remainder of the ophthalmic examination reveals bilateral age-related nuclear sclerosis and a general physical examination is unremarkable.

Further diagnostic tests
- Laboratory tests – routine haematology, biochemistry and urine analysis are unremarkable.
- Thoracic radiography and abdominal ultrasonography – results are unremarkable.
- B-mode ocular ultrasound – this can help confirm the presence of an iris mass and aid in assessment of the posterior segment if the view through the pupil is obscured. High-frequency ultrasound biomicroscopy can provide precise details about the extent of the involvement of the uveal tract (*Ch. 8, case 3, Fig. 8.3d*).

Ultrasound is not performed in this cat because a detailed intraocular examination is possible and the additional information does not alter the management of the case.

Diagnosis
Based on the information available, a presumptive diagnosis of diffuse iris melanoma in the right eye, and benign melanosis in the left eye is made.

The features in the right eye which support this diagnosis are the mass effect within the iris, dyscoria, reduced pupil mobility, the change in iris texture and thickening of the iris, as well as a raised IOP relative to the fellow eye. The features in the left eye which support this diagnosis are the absence of iris thickening, normal iris texture and the advanced age of the cat.

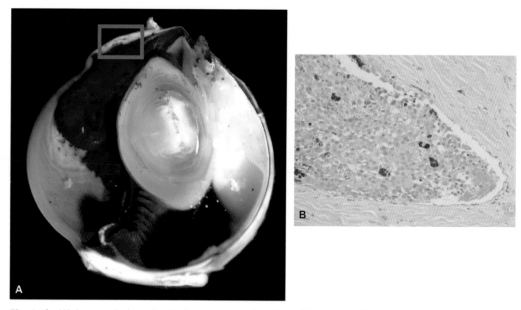

Fig. 9.3b (A) Gross pathology. Box indicates tumour invasion of the region of the scleral venous plexus. (B) Aggregate of neoplastic melanocytes plugging a vessel within the scleral venous plexus (H & E, ×400). Reproduced with permission from EJ Scurrell.

When characteristic features of diffuse iris melanoma are present, a biopsy is not warranted. When benign melanosis cannot be differentiated from early DIM on the basis of the ophthalmic examination, it would, in theory, be helpful to perform cytology or histopathology. Unfortunately, fine needle aspirates are unlikely to yield representative/diagnostic samples and an attempt to biopsy the iris tissue is likely to result in haemorrhage. Aqueous humour cytology has also been shown to provide unreliable information for the differentiation of the two conditions.

Treatment

Early enucleation is the treatment of choice for suspected DIM because of the risk of metastatic disease and can be justified on the basis of progressive hyperpigmentation, a pigmented mass, changes in the shape and mobility of the pupil, a perceived change in iris texture and an elevation in IOP. The right eye is removed by a routine transconjunctival enucleation and submitted for ocular histopathology. The histopathological diagnosis confirms the presence of advanced DIM with involvement of the filtration angle and invasion of the scleral venous plexus (Fig. 9.3b).

Prognosis

Enucleation in the early stage of DIM offers the best chance of survival. The prognosis is guarded in advanced disease because the metastatic rate is as high as 63% in some studies. Metastatic disease most frequently involves the liver and lungs but multiple organs can be affected. Disease latency is common and the clinical manifestation of metastatic disease can occur as late as one to three years following enucleation. Studies have described clinical and histopathological parameters to assist clinicians in the management of these cases. In one study, poor prognostic indicators included the presence of a high mitotic index, full thickness iris involvement and the presence of neoplastic cells

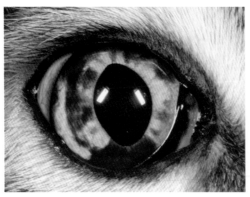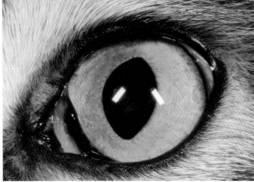

Fig. 9.3c Right and left eyes of a six-year-old domestic shorthaired cat. Multifocal areas of hyperpigmentation and an associated velveteen appearance are present in the right eye. Enucleation was advised and the histopathological diagnosis was early diffuse iris melanoma.

in the scleral venous plexus (Duncan & Peiffer, 1991). Another study correlated histopathological findings with survival times (Kalishman *et al.*, 1998). In this study, cats with tumour confined to the iris had survival times similar to the control group; cats with advanced tumour involvement of the iris, posterior iris epithelium, ciliary body and the scleral venous plexus had reduced survival times.

Discussion

Many veterinary pathologists believe that benign iridal melanosis in the cat is a pre-neoplastic lesion which may progress to malignancy in some cats. In benign melanosis, melanocytic proliferation is limited to the anterior iris surface and is seen clinically as hyperpigmentation. A change in melanocyte morphology associated with infiltration of the iris stroma is the hallmark of early DIM – this early change is only evident on histopathology. The rate of progression of DIM is impossible to predict as some lesions remain static, some slowly progress over years, and others rapidly progress over weeks to months. These factors make decisions about clinical management difficult – the dilemma for the clinician is deciding when to recommend enucleation.

The decisions made for this cat are straightforward because obvious clinical features of neoplasia are present. In cases where decision-making is less straightforward at initial presentation, regular monitoring is important, e.g. every three to six months.

For comparison, the eyes of two different cats are shown in Figs. 9.3c and 9.3d. Fig. 9.3c shows both eyes of a six-year-old female neutered domestic shorthaired cat with progressive iridal hyperpigmentation in the right eye over nine months. Enucleation was recommended on the basis of the rate of progression, a velveteen appearance observed with slit-lamp biomicroscopy, and unilaterality (benign melanosis is typically bilateral and more common in older cats). The histopathological diagnosis was early DIM.

Fig. 9.3d is from a three-year-old female neutered domestic shorthaired cat with progressive unilateral iris hyperpigmentation in the right eye over two years. Although the clinical presentation of this cat is similar to the cat in Fig. 9.3c, monitoring rather than enucleation was recommended on the basis of the slow rate of progression and the normal iris texture with slit-lamp biomicroscopy.

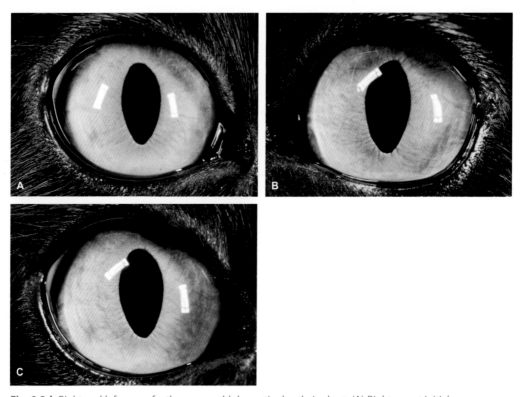

Fig. 9.3d Right and left eyes of a three-year-old domestic shorthaired cat. (A) Right eye at initial presentation. (B) Left eye appears normal. (C) Right eye two years later – progressive iridal hyperpigmentation. Monitoring was advised on the basis of the absence of any other clinical signs.

References and further reading

Duncan DE, Peiffer RL (1991) Morphology and prognostic indicators of anterior melanomas in cats. *Prog Vet Comp Ophthalmol*, **1**, 25–32.

Kalishman JB, Chappell RJ, Flood LA, Dubielzig RR (1998) A matched observational study of survival in cats with enucleation due to diffuse iris melanoma. *Vet Ophthalmol*, **1**(1), 25–29.

See Appendix 2.

History

A 4-year-old male neutered domestic longhaired cat is presented with a six-month history of a colour change in the right eye. He is an indoor/outdoor cat and has received routine vaccinations and regular anthelmintic treatment up until the last year.

Questions

1. Describe the abnormalities and pertinent normal features in Figs. 9.4a, b and c which show the appearance at presentation and one month later (see legends).
2. What differential diagnoses should be considered for this presentation?
3. What tests could you perform to make the diagnosis?

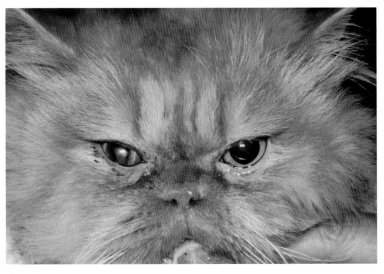

Fig. 9.4a

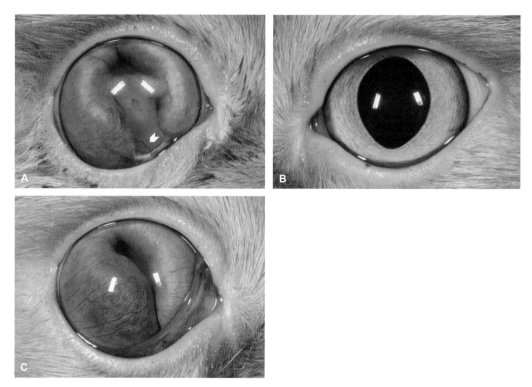

Fig. 9.4b Frontal view. (A) Right eye at presentation. (B) Left eye at presentation. (C) Right eye one month later.

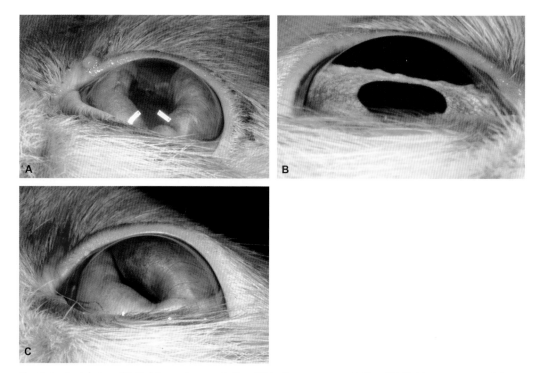

Fig. 9.4c Aerial view. (A) Right eye at presentation. (B) Left eye at presentation. (C) Right eye one month later.

Answers

1. What the figures show

Fig. 9.4a Left eye – there is a slight serous discharge. Right eye – there is a dried mucoid discharge, dyscoria and leukocoria because of a cataract.

Fig. 9.4b (frontal view) and **Fig. 9.4c** (aerial view) of both eyes: The left eye is normal. Right eye – there is gross distortion and generalised darkening of the iris with anterior displacement of iris tissue; this is most marked in the lateral and medial regions of the iris. The pupil is secluded and there is a poorly defined, scintillating corneal opacity (corneal lipidosis). The iris abnormalities in the right eye are more pronounced one month later, consistent with a progressive condition (Fig. 9.4b, C and 9.4c, C). The Purkinje images are normal.

2. Differential diagnoses

Given the appearance of the right eye, the following differential diagnoses should be considered:

- **Iris bombé** This is an anterior displacement or bowing of the iris caused by the circumferential formation of posterior synechiae as a result of anterior uveitis. The normal forward flow of aqueous humour from the ciliary body through the pupil towards the filtration angle is obstructed by adhesions. This leads to an accumulation of aqueous humour in the posterior chamber and the development of glaucoma.
- **Primary intraocular neoplasia**
  - **Diffuse iris melanoma (DIM)** This is the most common primary intraocular neoplasm in the cat and typically presents as a unilateral progressive hyperpigmentation of the iris over months to years. Hyperpigmentation can occur as a single area on the anterior surface of the iris or as multiple areas which become confluent with time. The earliest clinical sign of DIM is iridal hyperpigmentation, followed by a subtle velveteen change in the iris surface texture, iris thickening, dyscoria, reduced pupil mobility, pigment within the aqueous humour, and clinical signs of anterior uveitis; the presence of secondary glaucoma is consistent with advanced disease.
  - **Feline post-traumatic ocular sarcoma** This is an uncommon but highly malignant neoplasm, usually associated with a previous history of ocular trauma and lens injury. The clinical presentation is unilateral and can include signs of chronic uveitis, glaucoma, intraocular haemorrhage and a white/pink mass in the posterior segment of the eye.
  - **Iridociliary epithelial tumour (adenoma, adenocarcinoma)** These tumours arise from pigmented or non-pigmented cells of the iris or ciliary body and typically appear as a non-pigmented mass within the pupil or at the iris root. They are uncommon in the cat.
- **Lymphoma** Lymphoma is the most common metastatic intraocular tumour in the cat. It can appear as anterior uveitis, or a pink/white mass in the anterior chamber or both. In contrast to the dog, the majority of cats present with a nodular iris mass rather than with diffuse iris thickening. Although ocular lymphoma in the cat is generally considered to be a manifestation of multisystemic disease, primary ocular lymphoma is also suspected to occur. Aqueous humour cytology is frequently diagnostic as the tumour exfoliates cells readily.
- **Metastatic neoplasia** Neoplasia can metastasise haematogenously to the eye from local or distant sites or can invade the eye by direct local extension. Bilateral ocular involvement is characteristic of metastatic neoplasia, in contrast to the unilateral occurrence of primary ocular neoplasia. The uveal tract is a predilection site for haematogenous spread and metastatic neoplasia is consequently associated with uveitis and secondary glaucoma. Gross observation of metastatic neoplasia is often not possible because a mass lesion does not necessarily occur. Lymphoma is the most common secondary neoplasm in the eye; other examples include mammary gland adenocarcinoma, transitional cell carcinoma, haemangiosarcoma and osteosarcoma.

3. Appropriate diagnostic tests

- Ocular reflexes
  - Pupillary light reflex – positive direct and negative consensual OS, negative direct and consensual OD
  - Dazzle reflex – positive OS, negative OD
- Vision assessment
  - Menace response – positive OS, negative OD
  - Visual placing and tracking reflexes – positive OS, negative OD

In this cat, these results suggest that the right eye is blind. There is also a problem with pupil mobility in the right eye.

- Examination with a focal light source – in the right eye there is anterior displacement of the iris resulting in the obliteration of the anterior chamber and direct contact between the iris and the corneal endothelium. Slit-lamp biomicroscopy identifies a blood vessel extending from the iris at six o'clock, across the edge of the pupil and onto the anterior lens capsule (arrow, Fig. 9.4b, A).
- Schirmer test test – 10 mm/min OU
- Fluorescein dye – negative staining OU
- Tonometry – IOP 17 mmHg OS, 22 mmHg OD at initial presentation; 17 mmHg OS, 33 mmHg OD one month later. This is consistent with glaucoma in the right eye.

The remainder of the ophthalmic examination reveals no additional abnormalities and a general physical examination is unremarkable.

Further diagnostic tests

- Laboratory tests – routine haematology and biochemistry, urine analysis and serological tests for common infectious agents for a cat in north Europe (*Toxoplasma gondii*, FeLV, FIV and FIP) are performed to screen for systemic signs of uveitis or neoplasia. No abnormalities are found.
- B-mode ocular ultrasound – this reveals a hyperechoic area involving the posterior aspect of the lens and the anterior region of the vitreous humour, as well as a hyperechoic lens which is consistent with the cataract (Fig. 9.4d). Curvilinear hyperechoic structures in the anterior chamber

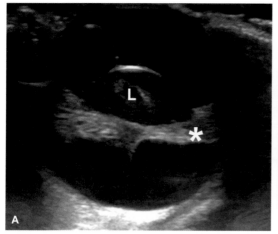
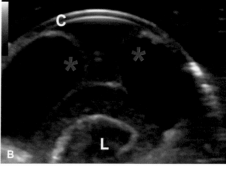

Fig. 9.4d B-mode ultrasound image of the right eye. (A) The lens is hyperechoic, consistent with a cataract; there is diffuse hyperechoic material within the anterior vitreous (white asterix), consistent with hyalitis. (B) Anterior displacement of the iris leaflets (blue asterix) in the anterior chamber. C, cornea; L, lens.

extend from the anterior surface of the lens to the corneal endothelium. This appearance is consistent with the anterior displacement of the iris leaflets observed in Figs. 9.4b and 9.4c.

- Thoracic radiography and abdominal ultrasound – these tests are performed to screen for systemic disease or neoplasia. Results are unremarkable.

Diagnosis

Based on the information available, a clinical diagnosis of iris bombé, cataract and glaucoma secondary to anterior uveitis in the right eye is made. The initiating cause of the uveitis is not identified but based on the absence of uveitis in the contralateral eye, the good general health of the cat, and the unremarkable results of the screening tests for systemic disease, lymphoplasmacytic uveitis or uveitis secondary to trauma are considered to be the most likely causes.

Treatment

Treatment options include symptomatic medical management for uveitis and secondary glaucoma, or enucleation *(Ch. 7, case 2)*. Medical therapy could include topical steroid therapy, e.g. 1% prednisolone acetate, and topical anti-glaucoma therapy, e.g. 2% dorzolamide, with or without 0.5% timolol maleate (Rainbow & Dziezyc, 2003; Dietrich *et al.*, 2007).

However, in this case the eye is considered to be irreversibly blind and a potential source of discomfort and so enucleation is elected. The right eye is removed by a routine transconjunctival procedure and submitted for ocular histopathology. The histopathological diagnosis confirms the presence of chronic low-grade lymphoplasmacytic uveitis, hyalitis, cataract and iris bombé – most probably the result of trauma (Fig. 9.4e).

> All enucleated globes should be submitted for ocular histopathology. For routine diagnostic purposes, fixation of the globe in 10% formalin is generally appropriate, although confirmation with the selected laboratory is recommended. Prior to fixation, as much excess extraocular tissue as possible should be removed, and the optic nerve should be left as long as possible.

Prognosis

The prognosis for the survival of this cat is excellent because neoplasia is excluded by histopathology. As the cause of the uveitis is presumed to be traumatic, the prognosis for the contralateral eye

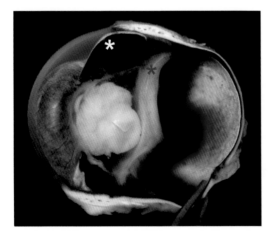

Fig. 9.4e Gross specimen of the right eye showing iris bombé (white asterix), cataract and opaque material within the anterior vitreous humour which represents chronic inflammation (hyalitis) (blue asterix). Reproduced with permission from EJ Scurrell.

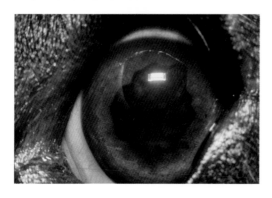

Fig. 9.4f Left eye of a dog with dyscoria caused by multiple posterior synechiae as a result of chronic anterior uveitis.

is considered to be good. However, monitoring is recommended because causes other than trauma have not been absolutely excluded.

Discussion

Iris bombé can mimic the appearance of anterior uveal neoplasia and as such require investigation. Ocular ultrasound can be beneficial to confirm that the abnormal appearance is the result of displacement rather than thickening of the iris.

Synechia formation is an indication of the severity or chronicity of anterior uveitis; it results from the presence of inflammatory cells and fibrin which facilitate the formation of adhesions between the pupil margin and the lens (posterior synechiae) or, less commonly, between the anterior iris and the cornea (anterior synechiae). A typical clinical example of anterior synechiae formation is in association with penetrating corneal trauma. Posterior synechiae are often focal and as a result only partially restrict mobility of the pupil, resulting in dyscoria (Fig. 9.4f). Iris bombé only occurs when the posterior synechiae formation is so extensive that the entire circumference of the pupil is involved, resulting in obstruction to the normal flow of the aqueous humour through the pupil.

Medical treatment for feline glaucoma has limited documented success – Blocker & van der Woerdt (2001) reported a 58% success rate in a retrospective study of 82 cats. This is most likely due to a combination of factors, including the fact that cats often present with chronic disease and the limited efficacy of available anti-glaucoma drugs in the cat. Some of the topical anti-glaucoma drugs that are widely used in the dog are ineffective in the cat. For example, topical prostaglandin agents are highly effective in acute primary canine glaucoma *(Ch. 6, case 2)* but are generally ineffective in the cat (Studer *et al.*, 2000; Regnier *et al.*, 2006). Dorzolamide and brinzolamide are topical carbonic anhydrase inhibitors that are frequently used in the management of canine glaucoma – although dorzolamide is effective in the cat (Rainbow & Dziezyc, 2003), brinzolamide is not (Gray *et al.*, 2003).

References and further reading

Blocker T & van der Woerdt A (2001) The feline glaucomas: 82 cases (1995–1999). *Vet Ophthalmol*, **4** (2), 81–85.

Czederpiltz JM, La Croix NC, van der Woerdt A, Bentley E, Dubielzig RR, Murphy CJ, *et al.* (2005) Putative aqueous humor misdirection syndrome as a cause of glaucoma in cats: 32 cases (1997–2003). *J AmVet Med Assoc*, **227**, 1434–1441.

Dietrich UM, Chandler MJ, Cooper T, Vidyashankar A, Chen G (2007) Effects of topical 2% dorzolamide hydrochloride alone and in combination with 0.5% timolol maleate on intraocular pressure in normal feline eyes. *Vet Ophthalmol*, **10**, (Suppl 1), 95–100.

Rainbow ME, Dziezyc J (2003) Effects of twice daily application of 2% dorzolamide on intraocular pressure in normal cats. *Vet Ophthalmol*, **6** (2), 147–150.

Regnier A, Lemagne C, Ponchet A, Cazolot G, Concordet D, Gelatt KN (2006) Ocular effects of topical 0.03% bimatoprost solution in normotensive feline eyes. *Vet Ophthalmol*, **9** (1), 39–43.

Studer ME, Martin CL, Stiles J (2000) Effects of 0.005% latanoprost solution on intraocular pressure in healthy dogs and cats. *Am J Vet Res*, **61** (10), 1220–1224.

See Appendix 2.

CHAPTER 10

The Abnormal Pupil

Introduction

The pupil is the window to the posterior segment of the eye. The iris sphincter muscle constricts the pupil to control the amount of light entering the eye and is under parasympathetic control in mammals. Sympathetic innervation of the iris provides constant antagonism to the iris sphincter muscle via the dilator muscle.

Abnormalities of the pupil usually involve changes in shape and size, and these are easiest to detect if a tapetal reflection is visible through the pupil. Pupil abnormalities are frequently the result of neuro-ophthalmic disorders and can be difficult to diagnose.

Small Animal Ophthalmology: What's Your Diagnosis? First Edition. Heidi Featherstone, Elaine Holt.
© 2011 by Heidi Featherstone and Elaine Holt. Published 2011 by Blackwell Publishing Ltd.

History

A 2-year-old female neutered English Springer Spaniel is presented with an acute onset of lethargy and anorexia, as well as an abnormal left eye. To the owner, the left eye appears to be smaller or more closed than the right eye but there is no apparent ocular discomfort. The dog has received routine vaccinations and regular anthelmintic treatment.

Questions

1. Describe the abnormalities and pertinent normal features in Figs. 10.1a and b.
2. What differential diagnoses should be considered for this presentation?
3. What tests could you perform to determine the specific diagnosis?

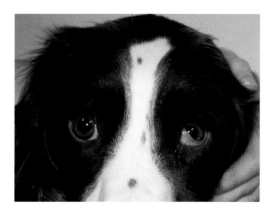

Fig. 10.1a

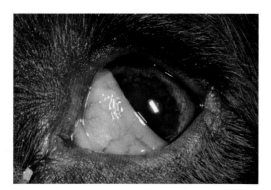

Fig. 10.1b

Answers

1. What the figures show

Figs. 10.1a and b The right eye appears normal. There is a relative anisocoria (OS < OD). Left eye – there is a scant, seromucoid discharge at the medial canthus. The palpebral fissure is smaller than in the right eye. There is ptosis of the lateral upper eyelid, enophthalmos (or possibly microphthalmos), protrusion and hyperaemia of the TEL.

2. Differential diagnoses

Given the appearance of the left eye, the following conditions/causes should be considered:

- **Horner's syndrome** This syndrome occurs when there is interruption to the sympathetic innervation of the eye and adnexa. The sympathetic pathway to the eye is a two-neuron system, which is controlled by higher centres of the autonomic nervous system in the brain. The pathway involves the brain, spinal cord, thorax, and eye. The pre-ganglionic axons synapse with the post-ganglionic axons in the cranial cervical ganglion (adjacent to the tympanic bulla). The post-ganglionic axons supply the smooth muscles of the peri-orbita, Muller's muscle of the upper and lower eyelids, and the iris dilator muscle. A lesion anywhere along this sympathetic pathway results in the clinical signs of Horner's syndrome – ptosis, enophthalmos, miosis, and TEL protrusion.

> Ptosis of the upper eyelid is a classic sign of Horner's syndrome but reverse ptosis or elevation of the lower eyelid may also be present because there is sympathetic innervation to the muscles in the lower eyelid as well as the upper eyelid. Ptosis and enophthalmos cause the palpebral fissure to be narrower or smaller than normal. Conjunctival hyperaemia is a less obvious sign of Horner's syndrome and is a result of local vasodilation. A mild ocular discharge is often seen in Horner's syndrome but is not considered to be part of the syndrome – it occurs because of reduced tear drainage as a result of the change in eye position.

- **Anterior uveitis** Inflammatory mediators cause painful spasm of the iris and ciliary body muscles, resulting in miosis. Ocular discomfort can also lead to blepharospasm and globe retraction by the retractor bulbi muscles. The clinical signs of anterior uveitis include miosis, enophthalmos, narrowed palpebral fissure and TEL protrusion.
- **Ocular surface pain** The cornea is innervated by the ophthalmic branch of the trigeminal nerve. Corneal stimulation can cause a reflex mediated by substance P. This axonal reflex can cause reflex uveitis and globe retraction by the retractor bulbi muscle. Globe retraction causes enophthalmos and passive TEL protrusion. The reflex uveitis appears as conjunctival hyperaemia, miosis, and TEL protrusion. Examples of causes of ocular surface pain include corneal ulceration, entropion and severe keratoconjunctivitis sicca.
- **Small globe** A small eye is recessed in the orbit compared to a normal sized eye. This results in passive TEL protrusion. Causes of a small globe include microphthalmos, nanophthalmos and phthisis bulbi *(Ch. 1, case 2)*. Microphthalmos can occur alone or in conjunction with multiple ocular defects including iris hypoplasia – the latter can result in miosis because of hypoplasia of the iris sphincter muscle.
- **Reduced volume of orbital tissue** This may cause the eye to be recessed in the orbit, resulting in TEL protrusion. Causes include dehydration, weight loss (reduction in orbital fat) and fibrosis of orbital tissues following orbital inflammation and surgery.
- **Space-occupying orbital lesion** An increase in the volume of orbital tissue, e.g. orbital mass, results in exophthalmos and TEL protrusion *(Ch. 1, case 3)*. A space-occupying lesion involving

the anterior orbit may push the eye caudally, causing enophthalmos and TEL protrusion e.g. local extension of a nasal tumour.

3. Appropriate diagnostic tests

- Ocular reflexes
  - PLR – direct and consensual positive OU. The anisocoria is more pronounced in scotopic conditions because the right pupil dilates normally while the left pupil remains small.
  - Dazzle reflex – positive OU
  - Palpebral reflex – present OU
  - Vestibulo-ocular reflex – present OU
- Menace response – positive OU

In this dog, these results suggest a lesion in the efferent pathway of the PLR in the left eye.

> If anisocoria is present, and is suspected to be caused by a neurological problem, it is important to establish which pupil is abnormal. The pupils should be assessed in both ambient light (photopic conditions) and in a darkened room (scotopic conditions). Assuming that no other ocular abnormalities are present (e.g. iris atrophy), some simple rules can be applied:
> - a normal pupil should dilate in the dark
> - a normal pupil should constrict with a bright light source
> - Horner's syndrome is likely to be present if the anisocoria is more pronounced in scotopic conditions (i.e. the difference in pupil size is more obvious in the dark).

- Examination with a bright focal light source – in both eyes, this reveals that the anterior chamber is normal with respect to depth and transparency, and the cornea is normal with respect to transparency and diameter. Assessment of corneal diameter is a useful indication of the size of the eye, e.g. corneal diameter is increased with buphthalmos (*Ch. 1, case 1*) and decreased with microphthalmos or phthisis bulbi (*Ch. 1, case 2*).
- Fluorescein dye – negative staining OU
- Tonometry – IOP 15 mmHg OU

There is no change in the position of the TEL in the left eye after administration of a topical anaesthetic. Retropulsion of both eyes is unremarkable. The remainder of the ophthalmic examination reveals no additional abnormalities. A general physical examination reveals reduced lung sounds on both sides of the chest; the external ear canals are normal. The remainder of the neurological assessment is unremarkable.

> Application of a topical anaesthetic agent will rapidly anaesthetise the ocular surface and can be helpful to determine whether TEL protrusion secondary to enophthalmos is because of ocular surface pain.

Further diagnostic tests

In order to help localise and identify the lesion further, the following additional diagnostic tests are performed:

Topical phenylephrine can be used to help confirm a diagnosis of Horner's syndrome. It can also help to determine the location of the lesion (see Discussion).

- Pharmacological testing – following one drop of topical 1% phenylephrine OU, the TEL protrusion in the left eye resolves within 5 min; the right eye is unaffected. After 40 min, the left pupil dilates to a greater extent than the right pupil (Fig. 10.1c). This result suggests that the miosis in the left eye is caused by a pre-ganglionic lesion in the sympathetic innervation of the iris dilator muscle.
- Radiography – thoracic radiography to assess the cervical and thoracic spinal cord and thorax reveals a large mediastinal mass.
- Ultrasonography – thoracic ultrasonography reveals a large mass of mixed echogenicity occupying the cranial mediastinum (Fig. 10.1d).
- CT – this is performed to evaluate further the extent of the lesion identified with radiography and ultrasound, as well as to determine if biopsy or surgical intervention is possible. CT examination of the thorax confirms the presence of a large mass in the dorsal aspect of the cranial mediastinum; the mass extends caudally to the level of the heart base, and displaces the intrathoracic trachea to the right side. This is consistent with the radiographic and ultrasonographic findings (Fig. 10.1e).

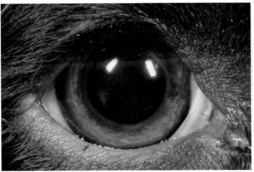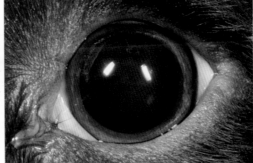

Fig. 10.1c Forty minutes after the topical administration of one drop of 1% phenyephrine to each eye – the left pupil is more dilated than the right pupil.

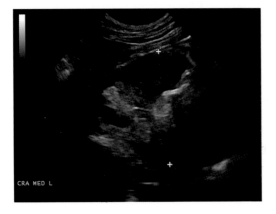

CRA MED L

Fig. 10.1d Ultrasound scan of thorax. Large mixed echoic mass in the cranial mediastinum.

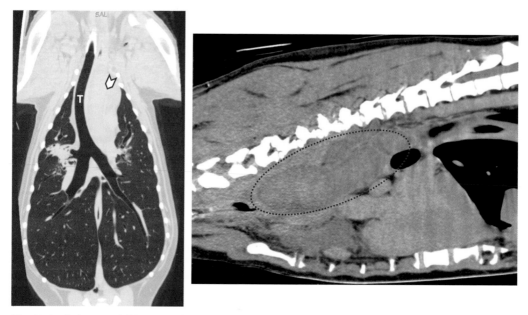

Fig. 10.1e Reformatted CT images. There is a large mass (arrow, dotted outline) in the dorsal aspect of the cranial mediastinum, extending caudally to the level of the heartbase and displacing the intrathoracic trachea (T) to the right side.

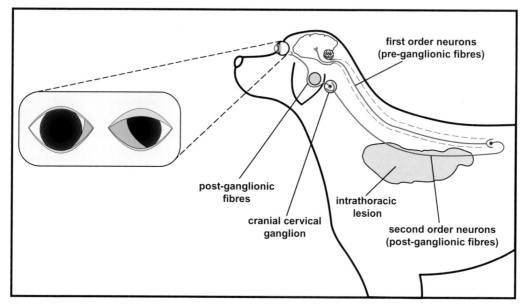

Diagram 10.1 Schematic representation of Horner's syndrome in this dog. The intrathoracic lesion affects second order pre-ganglionic fibres on the left side, resulting in Horner's syndrome in the left eye. Illustration by S Scurrell.

Diagnosis

Based on the information available, a diagnosis of pre-ganglionic Horner's syndrome in the left eye secondary to an intrathoracic mass is made (Diagram 10.1).

Treatment

The treatment of Horner's syndrome depends on the location and cause of the lesion. Most cases of Horner's syndrome in the dog are post-ganglionic and idiopathic although otitis media is often presumed to be the underlying cause. Symptomatic treatment with topical phenylephrine is advocated by some authors to relieve clinical signs in the short-term. Pre-ganglionic lesions, although less common, are more likely to require surgical intervention. In this dog, biopsies of the mediastinal mass are non-diagnostic and a left lateral thoracotomy is performed. Further histopathology reveals a haemangiosarcoma and the dog is subsequently euthanised.

Prognosis

The prognosis for a dog with Horner's syndrome depends on the cause and the location of the lesion. In general, post-ganglionic lesions have a better prognosis than pre-ganglionic lesions.

Discussion

The sympathetic pathway to the eye is controlled by higher centres of the autonomic nervous system in the brain. Efferent fibres leave the brain and travel along the cervical spinal cord to synapse on pre-ganglionic cell bodies located in the grey column of the first three thoracic spinal cord segments. The axons of these pre-ganglionic cell bodies exit the spinal cord as part of the spinal nerves and join the thoracic sympathetic trunk to continue towards the cranial cervical ganglion located ventromedial to the tympanic bulla. Within the cranial cervical ganglion, the axons synapse on post-ganglionic cell bodies from which post-ganglionic sympathetic axons pass rostrally on the external surface of the tympanic bulla before being distributed by the ophthalmic branch of the trigeminal nerve to supply the smooth muscles of the peri-orbita, Muller's muscle of the eyelid (upper and lower), and the iris dilator muscle. As well as playing a role in pupil size, sympathetic tone has a role in eyelid opening and influences the position of the eye within the orbit. A lesion anywhere along this sympathetic pathway results in Horner's syndrome.

Pharmacological testing is simple to perform but the results are not always reliable and should be interpreted with caution and in conjunction with other diagnostic tests. The underlying theory requires a detailed understanding of neuroanatomy and neurophysiology. Pharmacological testing is based on the 'law of denervation hypersensitivity'. This applies to both the sympathetic and para-sympathetic systems. Loss of autonomic innervations causes muscle fibres to become sensitised to cholinergic and adrenergic agents. Post-ganglionic lesions have a greater sensitivity to topically applied agents than pre-ganglionic lesions. Testing is employed to confirm that an ocular abnormality is neurological and can also aid in the localisation of the lesion. Several different drugs are described as being able to confirm and locate a Horner's lesion, but phenylephrine is most commonly used in veterinary medicine because of its availability. Phenylephrine is a direct-acting sympathomimetic agent that causes a normal pupil to dilate slowly (within two hours, depending on the concentration). In an eye with Horner's syndrome, the denervated sensitised smooth muscles of the iris and adnexa respond to low concentrations of phenylephrine more rapidly than a normal eye. The timing of a response to topical phenylephrine depends on the concentration of the drug applied – in general, a Horner's pupil will dilate more rapidly than a normal pupil, and a post-ganglionic lesion will cause a more rapid dilation of the pupil (<20 min) than a pre-ganglionic lesion (>40 min). Phenylephrine will also cause the TEL to return to its normal position; this generally occurs before a change in pupil size occurs.

The appearance of some common ophthalmic conditions is similar to Horner's syndrome, e.g. anterior uveitis. Although pharmacological testing has its limitations, it can be helpful to confirm that the ocular abnormality is neurological rather than ophthalmic in nature. It is probably for this reason that ophthalmologists often use pharmacological testing and neurologists do only rarely.

References and further reading

de Lahunta A & Glass E (2009) *Veterinary Neuroanatomy and Clinical Neurology*, 3rd edn. Saunders Elsevier, St Louis, Missouri, USA.

Penderis J (2004) Disorders of eyes and vision. In: *BSAVA Manual of Canine and Feline Neurology*, (eds S. Platt, N. Olby), 3rd edn. pp 144–145. British Small Animal Veterinary Association, Gloucester, UK.

Thomson HS (2003) The Pupil. In: *Alder's Physiology of the Eye*, (ed. WM Hart Jr), 9th edn. pp 434–437. Mosby-Year Book, USA.

See Appendix 2.

History

A 10-year-old female neutered domestic shorthaired cat is presented with a four-week history of a change in the appearance of the left eye and lethargy. The cat has received routine vaccinations and regular anthelmintic treatment, and is an indoor/outdoor cat.

Questions

1. Describe the abnormalities and pertinent normal features in Fig. 10.2a.
2. What differential diagnoses should be considered for this presentation?
3. What tests could you perform to make the diagnosis?

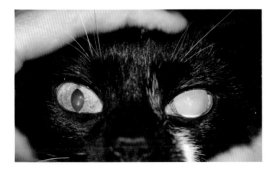

Fig. 10.2a

Answers

1. What the figure shows
Fig. 10.2a Left eye – the pupil is markedly dilated. Right eye – there is a focal area of iris pigmentation at the 12 o'clock position, an incidental finding in this cat (*see Ch. 9, case 3 for causes of iris pigmentation in the cat*).

2. Differential diagnoses
Given the clinical diagnosis of anisocoria, the following conditions/explanations should be considered for the left eye:

- **Oculomotor nerve lesion** Post-ganglionic parasympathetic fibres travel with the oculomotor nerve to the iris sphincter muscle and are responsible for contraction of the pupil (miosis). The oculomotor nerve also supplies somatic efferent fibres to four of the extraocular muscles (dorsal, medial, and ventral recti and ventral oblique) and the levator palpebrae superioris muscle (upper eyelid); these muscles are involved in eye movement and elevation of the upper eyelid, respectively. A lesion involving the oculomotor nucleus or nerve can cause internal ophthalmoplegia (paralysis of the iris and ciliary body muscles) which is manifested as ipsilateral mydriasis (Adie's pupil). Other clinical signs are ventrolateral strabismus and upper ptosis in the affected eye.
- **Cavernous sinus syndrome (orbital fissure syndrome)** The oculomotor nerve passes through the cavernous sinus (paired sinuses at the base of the skull) and the orbital fissure (in the caudal wall of the orbit) and can therefore be affected by lesions in both areas. The trochlear nerve, abducens nerve and ophthalmic and mandibular branches of the trigeminal nerve, also pass through these areas. The clinical presentation of cavernous sinus syndrome reflects the involvement of multiple nerves. It is characterised by internal ophthalmoparesis/ophthalmoplegia (fixed, dilated pupil), decreased or absent corneal sensation and an inability to retract the globe. This syndrome is most commonly caused by neoplasia but, in the cat, can be secondary to inflammatory disease.
- **Retinal disease** Generalised retinal pathology causes mydriasis in the affected eye and anisocoria if the disease is unilateral, e.g. unilateral retinal detachment secondary to systemic hypertension. If the disease is extensive enough to cause marked mydriasis, the PLR and vision will also be affected.
- **Optic nerve disease** A lesion of the optic nerve will cause mydriasis in the affected eye and anisocoria if the disease is unilateral. Optic nerve disorders are uncommon in the cat and include optic nerve atrophy following traumatic ocular proptosis, glaucoma, retinal degeneration, neoplasia (meningioma). As with extensive retinal disease, the PLR and vision will also be affected.

Mydriasis is usually greater with a lesion involving the efferent pathway of the PLR than with a lesion involving the afferent pathway. Complete unilateral lesions of the retina and/or the optic nerve (afferent pathway) usually result in partial rather than complete mydriasis. This is because parasympathetic tone (which decreases pupil size) results from light stimulation of the contralateral eye.

- **Abnormalities of the iris**
  - **Iris atrophy** Atrophy of the iris sphincter and dilator muscles causes mydriasis and a reduced PLR.
  - **Iris coloboma** A congenital abnormality which involves partial or complete absence of the iris tissue. Iris coloboma can result in mydriasis and a reduced PLR.

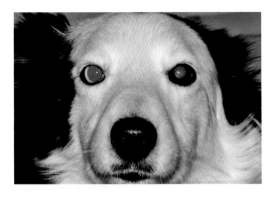

Fig. 10.2b Heterochromia iridis and associated anisocoria in a Border Collie. The left eye has a brown iris and a yellow tapetal reflection; the right eye has a blue iris and a red tapetal reflection (from a subalbinotic fundus) and a mild resting anisocoria (OS < OD). Reproduced with permission from J Mould.

- ○ **Heterochromia iridis** Unilateral heterochromia iridis can cause mydriasis. Anisocoria results because the pupil ipsilateral to the lighter coloured iris is larger than the contralateral pupil (Fig. 10.2b).
- ○ **Posterior synechiae** Adhesions between the iris and the anterior lens capsule can cause dyscoria and an immobile pupil; anisocoria will result if the lesion is unilateral.
- **Glaucoma** Unilateral mydriasis is an important and classic clinical sign of acute glaucoma. Mydriasis with glaucoma is presumed to be caused by damage to the optic nerve and retina and hypoxia of the iris musculature initially, and by iris atrophy in more advanced disease. In contrast to the dog (*Ch. 6, case 2*), glaucoma in cats tends to have an insidious onset and is often difficult to recognise. Additional clinical signs include buphthalmos, conjunctival and episcleral congestion, corneal oedema, mydriasis, and impaired or absent vision (*Ch.1, case 1*). It is therefore unusual for a cat with glaucoma to present with unilateral mydriasis alone. However 'aqueous humour misdirection syndrome' is a form of feline glaucoma that can cause unilateral (most commonly) or bilateral mydriasis. Aqueous humour misdirection syndrome (or ciliovitreolenticular block glaucoma) involves displacement of the iris-lens diaphragm which then appears convex and results in a shallow anterior chamber and raised intraocular pressure (Czederpiltz *et al.*, 2005).
- **Lens luxation** Miosis or mydriasis can result from lens dislocation depending on the presence of uveitis or glaucoma, as well as the position of the lens; dyscoria is also often present.
- **Drug-induced mydriasis** Topical administration of sympathomimetic or parasympatholytic agents will induce mydriasis in the treated eye (and to some extent in the contralateral eye, depending on the agent and the degree of systemic absorption of the drug).

3. Appropriate diagnostic tests

If anisocoria is present, and is suspected to be caused by a neurological problem, it is important to establish which pupil is abnormal. The pupils should be assessed in both ambient light (photopic conditions) and in a darkened room (scotopic conditions). Assuming that no other ocular abnormalities are present (e.g. iris atrophy), some simple rules can be applied:
- a normal pupil should dilate in the dark
- a normal pupil should constrict with a bright light source
- Horner's syndrome is likely to be present if the anisocoria is more pronounced in scotopic conditions (i.e. the difference in pupil size is more obvious in the dark)

- Ocular reflexes
  - Pupillary light reflex – negative direct and positive consensual OS (left to right eye), positive direct and negative consensual OD (right to left eye). Anisocoria (OS > OD) is present in both photopic and scotopic conditions but is less pronounced in the dark (because the right pupil dilates normally).
  - Dazzle reflex – positive OU
  - Palpebral reflex – positive OU
  - Corneal reflex – positive OU
  - Swinging flashlight test – negative OU
  - Vestibulo-ocular reflex – negative OS, positive OD. With cervical extension, the right eye moves ventrally (normal), but the left eye remains fixed in position (Fig. 10.2c). When the head is turned to the right side, the right eye moves in a medial direction (normal) but the left eye remains fixed in position (Fig. 10.2d). The finding in the left eye is consistent with external ophthalmoplegia (paralysis of the external ocular muscles).
- Vision testing
  - Menace response – positive OU
  - Visual placing and tracking reflexes – positive OU
  - Obstacle course – the results are considered to be unreliable as the cat is unwilling to move around the examination room.

In this cat, these findings suggest that the left eye has absent motility, the left pupil is abnormal and that the lesion involves the efferent pathway of the PLR.

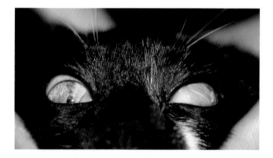

Fig. 10.2c Vestibulo-ocular reflex. During cervical extension, the right eye rotates in a ventral direction (normal) and the left eye remains fixed in position (abnormal).

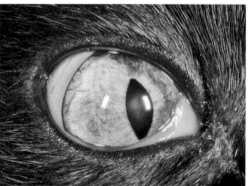 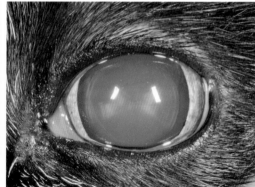

Fig. 10.2d Vestibulo-ocular reflex. When the head is turned to the right side, the right eye moves in a medial direction (normal) and the left eye remains fixed in position (abnormal).

The swinging flashlight test (SFT) can be helpful to determine if mydriasis is caused by a unilateral pre-chiasmal lesion (retina, optic nerve, or optic tract up to the level of the chiasm). To perform a SFT first assess the PLR in one eye, then shine the light source in the fellow eye; quickly move the light source back to the first eye, and then immediately back to the fellow eye. If the pupil in the fellow eye is seen to dilate rather than constrict in response to the light source, the SFT is said to be positive. This is known as a Marcus-Gunn pupil and is a pathognomonic clinical sign for a unilateral pre-chiasmal lesion.

- Pharmacological testing – following one drop of 1% pilocarpine in both eyes, both pupils constrict but the response is asymmetrical. The mydriatic left pupil constricts more rapidly (within 10 min) and to a greater extent than the right pupil (Fig. 10.2e). This result confirms that the mydriasis in the left eye is caused by a neurological problem but does not localise the lesion.
- Tonometry – IOP 18 mmHg OU

Pharmacological testing is simple to perform but the results can be unreliable and should be interpreted with caution. Physostigmine and pilocarpine are parasympathomimetic agents and are both used to assess an eye with a dilated pupil suspected of having an oculomotor nerve lesion (Adie's pupil).

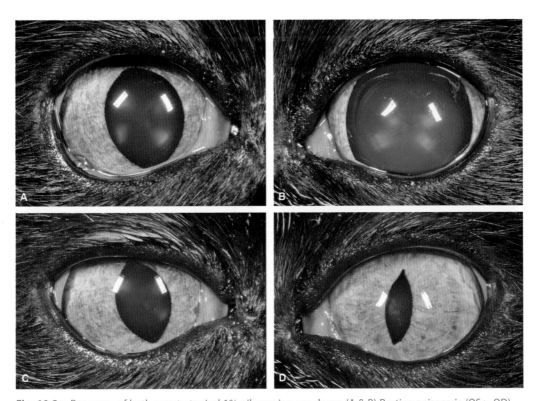

Fig. 10.2e Response of both eyes to topical 1% pilocarpine eye drops. (A & B) Resting anisocoria (OS > OD) before administration of pilocarpine. (C & D) Ten minutes following administration of pilocarpine: the abnormal left pupil constricts to a greater extent than normal right pupil, consistent with a parasympathetic lesion on the left side.

Retropulsion of both eyes is unremarkable. The remainder of the ophthalmic and neurological examination reveals no further abnormalities; a general physical examination is also unremarkable.

Further diagnostic tests

- Laboratory tests – routine haematology, biochemistry and urine analysis are recommended prior to general anaesthesia which is necessary for advanced imaging. All results are unremarkable.
- Forced duction test – this test helps to differentiate mechanical restriction from a neurological disorder in an eye with reduced motility. It can be performed in a conscious (active forced duction) or unconscious, anaesthetised animal (passive forced duction).

  A passive forced duction test is performed in this cat. The left eye is grasped with fine rat-toothed forceps close to the limbus and is freely moveable in all directions. This excludes the presence of mechanical restriction and suggests that the abnormal vestibulo-ocular reflex is the result of a neurological problem.
- MRI brain scan – the sagittal and transverse T2-weighted MRI images of the brain demonstrate a right-sided mass, 1 cm in diameter, ventral to the thalamus and causing a mild midline shift to the left (Fig. 10.2f). The appearance of the mass is consistent with a meningioma.

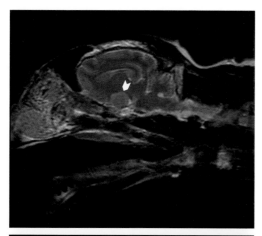

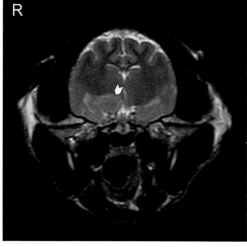

Fig. 10.2f MRI brain scans (sagittal and transverse T2-weighted images). There is a right-sided, 1-cm mass (arrow) ventral to the thalamus causing a mild midline shift to the left. The appearance of the lesion is consistent with a meningioma. Reproduced with permission from R Dennis, Animal Health Trust.

Diagnosis

Based on the information available, the diagnosis is internal and external ophthalmoplegia in the left eye secondary to an intracranial meningioma.

Treatment

Management options for intracranial meningiomas in the cat include corticosteroid therapy, radiotherapy and surgical excision. In contrast to the dog, adjunctive radiotherapy after surgical excision is not usually performed in the cat because the lesions are generally benign and progress extremely slowly. Systemic corticosteroid therapy may be beneficial if there is oedema surrounding the tumour, as it can temporarily improve demeanour and clinical signs in some cats. Surgery is not an option for the meningioma in this cat because of its location. A detailed discussion of the treatment options for meningioma is beyond the scope of this book.

Prognosis

Although meningiomas in the cat are slowly progressive, the prognosis for survival is guarded. At the time of writing there is very limited recent published information on the prognosis for survival in cats with meningiomas, which is in contrast to the dog (*Ch. 11, case 5*). Depending on the location, surgical excision of a cerebral meningioma is possible, and the reported median survival in the cat is 71% at 6 months, 66% at 1 year, and 50% at 2 years (Lori *et al.*, 2008).

Discussion

This case demonstrates the complexity of localising neurologic lesions affecting the pupil. In cats, a neurologic deficit which results in anisocoria is more frequently attributed to Horner's syndrome than to a lesion involving the oculomotor nerve.

See the 'Discussion' in case 1 of this chapter for more details on the principals of pharmacological testing. Physostigmine and pilocarpine are parasympathomimetic agents and both can be used in the pharmacological testing of an eye with a dilated pupil that is suspected to be caused by an oculomotor nerve lesion (Adie's pupil). Pilocarpine acts directly on the iris sphincter muscle, inducing miosis. A mydriatic pupil secondary to an oculomotor lesion will constrict faster and to a greater extent than a normal pupil (as occurred in this cat). The timing of the constriction depends on the concentration of drug used, e.g. 1% pilocarpine will cause a normal pupil to constrict within 20 min. Pilocarpine can confirm that the problem is neurological and can also differentiate between a neurological problem and a mechanical problem or pharmacological blockade (e.g. previous application of topical atropine). However, pilocarpine does not localise the lesion. Physostigmine has an indirect action because it requires an intact post-ganglionic neuron to induce miosis. Physostigmine will cause a normal pupil to constrict within 45–60 min but an Adie's pupil caused by a pre-ganglionic lesion will constrict more rapidly (<45 min). Physostigmine can be used both to confirm that the problem is neurological and to localise the lesion. If available, physostigmine should be used prior to pilocarpine, with an interval of at least 24 h between drugs. In the clinical setting, pharmacological testing is usually performed with pilocarpine only because physostigmine is not readily available.

Internal ophthalmoplegia refers to paralysis of the iris sphincter and ciliary body muscles and appears clinically as a fixed and dilated pupil. External ophthalmoplegia refers to paralysis of the extraocular muscles (innervated by oculomotor, trochlear and abducens nerves), and appears clinically as an eye that is unable to move in any direction. However, because the parasympathetic and motor nuclei of the oculomotor nerve lie adjacent to each other in the brain and their axons travel together within the oculomotor nerve, the most common clinical presentation is concurrent internal and external ophthalmoplegia, i.e. total ophthalmoplegia. For example, cavernous sinus syndrome results in total ophthalmoplegia (and reduced corneal sensation). The extraocular muscles are innervated by the oculomotor, trochlear and abducens nerves and so it is possible that a small degree of globe movement could be retained if only the oculomotor nerve is affected (partial external ophthalmoplegia). It is not usually possible to appreciate this clinically. Internal ophthalmoplegia can occur alone because the parasympathetic fibres along the medial side of the oculomotor nerve are superficial and more vulnerable to trauma. External ophthalmoplegia is most likely to occur when the lesion is central – this provides valuable diagnostic information which can aid with localisation.

References and further reading

Czederpiltz JM, La Croix NC, van der Woerdt A, *et al.* (2005) Putative aqueous humor misdirection syndrome as a cause of glaucoma in cats: 32 cases (1997–2003). *J Am Vet Med Assoc*, **227** (9), 1434–1441.

Thomson HS (2003) The Pupil. In: *Alder's Physiology of the Eye*, (ed. WM Hart, Jr), 9th edn, pp 429–434. Mosby-Year Book, USA.

Lori EG, Thacher C, Matthiesen DT, Joseph RJ (2008) Results of craniotomy for the treatment of cerebral meningioma in 42 cats. *Vet Surg*, **23** (2), 94–100.

Troxel MT, Vite CH, van Winkle TJ, *et al.* (2003) Feline intracranial neoplasia: retrospective review of 160 cases. *J Vet Intern Med*, **17**, 850–859.

See Appendix 2.

CHAPTER 11

The Blind Eye

Introduction

The visual pathway begins in the eye and terminates in the visual cortex of the brain. An abnormality anywhere along this pathway has the potential to impair vision and, if severe, to cause blindness. A thorough investigation into the cause of blindness requires assessment of retinal function, which may include electroretinography. Advanced imaging with MRI or CT is often necessary to assess optic nerve or central causes of vision loss. The onset of blindness in animals is often characterised as sudden or gradual. However, an owner's observations of a pet can be misleading, as an animal that has previously adapted well to slow but progressive vision loss can suddenly appear blind.

Small Animal Ophthalmology: What's Your Diagnosis? First Edition. Heidi Featherstone, Elaine Holt.
© 2011 by Heidi Featherstone and Elaine Holt. Published 2011 by Blackwell Publishing Ltd.

History

A seven-year-old female neutered English Cocker Spaniel is presented with a 12-month history of progressive visual impairment. The vision loss is most apparent during evening walks and the owner has also noticed that both eyes appear 'glazed'. The dog has received routine vaccinations and regular anthelmintic treatment and is otherwise clinically well.

Questions

1. Describe the abnormalities and pertinent normal features in Figs. 11.1a, b and c.
2. What differential diagnoses should be considered for this presentation?
3. What tests could you perform to make the diagnosis?

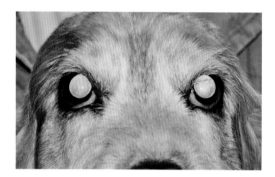

Fig. 11.1a Reproduced with permission from J Mould.

Fig. 11.1b

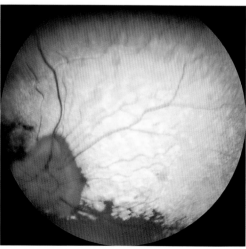

Fig. 11.1c

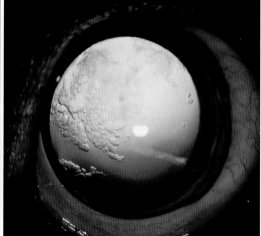

Answers

1. What the figures show
Fig. 11.1a Both eyes – the pupil is very dilated. The yellow tapetal reflection is slightly hazy.

Fig. 11.1b Fundic photograph. Left eye – there is marked tapetal hyperreflectivity, which appears as a homogeneous sheen, and attenuation of the retinal vasculature. The optic disc is pale and the venous circle is less prominent than expected – these changes are consistent with optic nerve atrophy. Similar changes are present in the right eye (not shown).

Fig. 11.1c Left eye – there are diffuse, irregular opacities and vacuoles (bubbles) in the lens, predominantly in the equatorial region. Similar changes are present in the right eye (not shown).

2. Differential diagnoses
Given the appearance of the bilateral fundic and lens abnormalities, the clinical diagnosis is advanced generalised retinal degeneration and early cataract formation. The following conditions should be considered:

- **Hereditary retinopathy**
  - **Progressive retinal degeneration (PRA)** This term refers to a group of hereditary retinal degenerations characterised by a primary defect in the photoreceptors in the neurosensory retina. Although the primary defects at the cellular level differ, the clinical signs are remarkably similar between the different forms of PRA. The most important clinical sign is visual impairment, which always ultimately leads to total blindness. As rod photoreceptors are usually affected before the cones, night blindness (nyctalopia) usually occurs before day blindness (hemeralopia). The age of onset and the rate of progression of the disease are different, depending on the breed. Secondary cataracts are common. The photoreceptor defect leads to atrophy of the neurosensory retina, which appears ophthalmoscopically as tapetal hyperreflectivity. This is followed by retinal vasculature attenuation and optic disc atrophy (pale optic disc with an indistinct venous circle). In advanced disease, there is a loss of pigment in the non-tapetal fundus which results in a patchy, mottled appearance called 'pavementing'.
  - **Retinal pigment epithelial dystrophy (RPED)** (formerly known as central progressive retinal degeneration) A hereditary retinal degeneration characterised by an abnormality in the retinal pigment epithelium (RPE). A light brown pigment accumulates within the RPE cells, causing hypertrophy, and subsequent degeneration of the overlying photoreceptors. The pigment is autofluorescent and is similar to ceroid and lipofuscin. RPED is characterised by progressive visual impairment, which may lead to blindness in some dogs. Vision tends to be better in low light levels and for moving objects in the distance; secondary cataracts are uncommon although they may occur in advanced cases. Ophthalmoscopically, RPED appears initially as multiple brown pigment spots in the central tapetal fundus; these pigment foci later become interspersed with areas of tapetal hyper-reflectivity (Fig. 11.1d). RPED is most frequently seen in the UK but is uncommon.
  - **Retinal dysplasia** Abnormal development of the retina, with proliferation of one or more of its elements. Although a hereditary cause of retinal dysplasia is most common, there are non-hereditary forms, e.g. those caused by viral infections and intra-uterine trauma. The typical fundoscopic appearance of retinal dysplasia is multiple greyish-white dots or linear steaks most prevalent in the central region of the retina; larger geographic lesions and retinal detachment may also occur. This is a congenital condition and is generally not associated with progressive visual impairment.
  - **Neuronal ceroid lipofuscinosis** A group of progressive neurodegenerative diseases characterised by brain and retinal atrophy because of an abnormal accumulation of autofluorescent

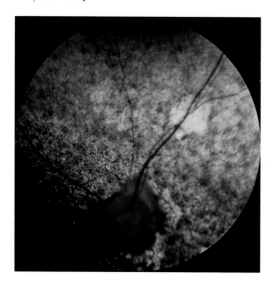

Fig. 11.1d Relatively advanced RPED in an English Cocker Spaniel. There are multiple brown pigment foci scattered throughout the tapetal fundus, interspersed with tapetal hyperreflectivity; there is also secondary attenuation of the retinal vasculature.

lipopigments in neurons. Cortical blindness is most common but the retina may be affected in some breeds.

- **Post-inflammatory retinal degeneration** Inflammation of the retina (retinitis) is usually secondary to inflammation from the adjacent choroid (chorioretinitis). Post-inflammatory retinal lesions appear as multifocal areas of tapetal hyperreflectivity and increased pigmentation. This is because of atrophy of the neurosensory retina and melanin proliferation in the RPE, respectively. Localised vascular attenuation may accompany the lesions. If the problem is bilateral, the appearance is usually different between eyes. If the initial inflammatory process is generalised, then diffuse retinal degeneration may occur.

- **Retinal degeneration following retinal detachment and subsequent reattachment** Retinal detachment almost always involves separation of the neurosensory retina from the underlying RPE on which it depends for normal function. This loss of structural integrity causes degeneration of the affected retina to begin within hours. Even if the retina subsequently reattaches, there will be a loss of function. If the detachment is extensive, the affected eye may subsequently be blind because of generalised retinal degeneration.

- **Retinal degeneration secondary to glaucoma** Glaucoma can lead to optic nerve damage alone or in addition to localised or generalised retinal degeneration. Localised retinal degeneration may be restricted to the peri-papillary area (tapetal hyperreflectivity around the optic disc) or appear as fan-shaped areas of degeneration radiating from the optic disc; these areas are known as 'watershed lesions'. In retinal degeneration secondary to glaucoma, the inner retinal layers are affected first, and more specifically, the retinal ganglion cell layer.

- **Nutritional retinopathy**
  - **Vitamin A deficiency** This can lead to nyctalopia but is clinically very rare in the dog.
  - **Vitamin E deficiency** Vitamin E is an antioxidant which maintains cell membrane stability and its deficiency can lead to pathologic changes within the retina, muscle, central nervous system and reproductive tract. The fundic changes in vitamin E deficiency and RPED are very similar and suggest that there may be a common aetiologic factor. This has been substantiated in the English Cocker Spaniel in which a familial primary vitamin E deficiency has been described.

- **Toxic retinopathy** Bilateral retinal degeneration has been documented to occur with some systemic drugs, e.g. ethambutol, azalide and closantel.

- **Light-induced retinopathy** Retinal degeneration can occur following prolonged exposure to light, e.g. indirect ophthalmoscopy, or from an operating microscope during intraocular surgery.
- **Retinopathy induced by radiation** Retinal damage can occur following radiation therapy for neoplasia involving regions of the head and neck.

3. Appropriate diagnostic tests

- Ocular reflexes
  - Pupillary light reflex – positive direct and consensual OU, albeit slow and incomplete
  - Dazzle reflex – positive but reduced OU
- Vision testing
  - Menace response – equivocal OU
  - Visual placing and tracking reflexes – results are unreliable
  - Obstacle course – this dog is able to navigate around large objects without hesitation in photopic conditions but there is marked hesitation in scotopic conditions.

In this dog, these findings suggest reduced vision in both eyes which is most pronounced in dim light.

- Examination with a focal light source – in both eyes, slit-lamp biomicroscopy identifies the lens opacities as vacuoles and localises them to the posterior cortex and the equator.
- Tonometry – IOP 17 mmHg OU
- Electroretinography – this is not indicated because retinal function will be decreased if diffuse retinal degeneration is visible on fundoscopic examination.
- Genetic testing – DNA-based tests are commercially available to identify many forms of PRA. Genetic testing can be helpful, particularly as the breeding age may be earlier than the onset of the disease. Most laboratories request either a blood sample or a cheek swab for a DNA-based test.

    Genetic testing is not performed in this dog because the breed, age, history and clinical presentation are considered classic for PRA.

The remainder of the ophthalmic examination reveals no further abnormalities and a general physical examination is unremarkable.

Diagnosis

Based on the information available, a diagnosis of PRA with secondary cataract is made; in the English Cocker Spaniel, this is more specifically termed progressive rod-cone degeneration (prcd).

Treatment

Currently, no treatment is available for PRA in the dog. The dog is an important animal model for inherited retinal degeneration in humans – potential therapeutic approaches are being investigated in animal models and in human clinical trials. These include gene therapy, retinal neuroprotection, retinal transplantation, stem cell therapy, retinal prostheses, and dietary supplementation.

Prognosis

PRA always leads to total blindness. However, most affected dogs cope well as the deterioration in vision is gradual (years in some breeds) and there is no associated ocular discomfort. Cataract surgery is contraindicated in dogs with PRA unless the cataracts are relatively advanced when the retina is only mildly affected – this situation is seen most commonly in the English Cocker Spaniel. In this breed a small number of affected dogs may benefit from cataract surgery to prolong vision, even if it is for a limited period because of progressive retinal degeneration.

Discussion

PRA in the dog can be simply divided into developmental and degenerative disease, and further subdivided on the basis of the cell type that is affected. The most common form of PRA is prcd, an autosomal recessive, late-onset retinal degeneration. First described in the 1980s, prcd is an allelic condition, i.e. the same gene is responsible for the disease in several different breeds. The specific defective gene for prcd has since been identified. Breeds affected with prcd include the Miniature and Toy Poodle, Labrador Retriever, and American and English Cocker Spaniel. Cataracts secondary to PRA are common – they are generally bilaterally symmetrical and occur when the retinal degeneration is advanced but there are some exceptions, e.g. English Cocker Spaniel. The cataract begins in the posterior cortex and extends into the equator and anterior cortex, ultimately forming a mature/complete cataract. Vacuoles in the equatorial region of the lens are a common finding in cataracts secondary to PRA. Lens vacuoles are bubble-like lesions that represent swelling of the lens fibres and are usually indicative of active cataract formation. Although a characteristic finding in dogs with PRA, lens vacuoles are also commonly seen in rapidly developing cataracts secondary to diabetes mellitus and trauma.

Further reading

See Appendix 2.

History

An 8-year-old female neutered cross-breed dog is presented with a history of acute vision loss over three to four days. The owner also reports that the dog is polydipsic and polyuric, subdued and has gained weight. The dog's general health has been unremarkable prior to the onset of this problem; she has received routine vaccinations and regular anthelmintic treatment.

Questions

1. Describe the abnormalities and pertinent normal features in Fig. 11.2a.
2. What differential diagnoses should be considered for this presentation?
3. What tests could you perform to make the diagnosis?

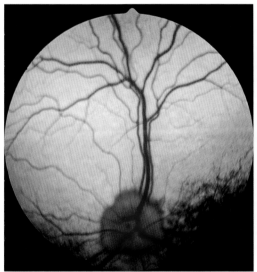 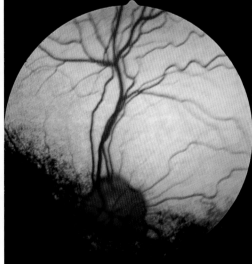

Fig. 11.2a

Answers

1. What the figure shows
Fig. 11.2a Fundic photograph. Both eyes – the optic disc is a slightly different shape in each eye because of pronounced myelination; this is a common and normal finding in the dog.

2. Differential diagnoses
Given the history of sudden onset blindness together with the normal appearance of the fundus in both eyes, the following conditions should be considered:

- **Sudden acquired retinal degeneration syndrome (SARDS)** A retinal disorder of unknown cause that results in sudden onset blindness in affected dogs. The clinical presentation is characterised by a sudden loss of vision over several days to weeks which may be associated with polydipsia, polyuria, polyphagia and weight gain. Any breed or cross-breed dog can be affected and most affected animals are middle-aged. The fundus initially appears normal but signs of retinal degeneration (tapetal hyperreflectivity, retinal vascular attenuation and optic disc atrophy) develop over several months. Electroretinography produces a 'flat-line' response, consistent with a lack of retinal function.
- **Optic neuritis** Inflammation of the optic nerve can affect the intraocular (at the level of the optic disc), intraorbital (retrobulbar) or central portion of the optic nerve. Optic neuritis can be unilateral or bilateral and typically causes a sudden loss of vision in the affected eye. The optic disc is swollen and raised; its margins may be blurred and haemorrhages may be present. However, if the intraocular portion of the nerve is unaffected, the fundus will appear normal. In contrast to SARDS, electroretinography is expected to be normal because retinal function is generally unaffected (*case 4, this chapter*).
- **Central blindness (amaurosis)** A lesion involving the central visual pathway can cause blindness. From the optic chiasm the optic tracts carry visual fibres which synapse within the lateral geniculate nucleus. Post-synaptic fibres then leave the lateral geniculate nucleus as the optic radiations, which terminate in the visual cortex of the cerebrum (lateral, caudal and medial aspects of the occipital lobe) (*case 5, this chapter*).
- **Immune-mediated retinitis (IMR)** A syndrome recently described by veterinary ophthalmologists at Iowa State University in the USA; the clinical appearance of dogs with IMR appears to be similar to that of SARDS. Investigations into the characterisation, diagnosis and treatment of this syndrome are on-going at the time of writing.

3. Appropriate diagnostic tests
- Ocular reflexes
  - Pupillary light reflex – negative direct and consensual OU
  - Dazzle reflex – negative OU
  - Vestibulo-oculocephalic reflex – positive OU
- Vision testing
  - Menace response – negative OU
  - Visual placing and tracking reflexes – negative OU
  - Obstacle course – the dog is unable to navigate around large objects in both photopic and scotopic conditions.

In this dog, these results are consistent with blindness in both eyes.

- Tonometry – IOP 17 mmHg OU
- Colorimetric PLR testing – a recently described simple and inexpensive method for assessing photoreceptor and retinal ganglion cell function. This test investigates the response of the PLR

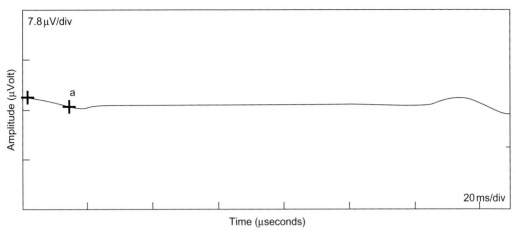

Fig. 11.2b Electroretinogram. Flat-line response confirms absent retinal function.

to a red and blue light stimulus. If retinal function is reduced or absent and the disease involves the photoreceptor layer and/or the retinal ganglion cell layer, e.g. SARDS or IMR, the PLR is positive with a blue light stimulus but negative with a red light stimulus.

In this dog, the direct and consensual PLR is negative with both the standard white light and red light stimuli, but positive with the blue light stimulus. This is consistent with a disease involving the photoreceptor layer and/or the retinal ganglion cell layer

- Electroretinography – flat-line response OU. This is consistent with absent retinal function in both eyes (Fig. 11.2b).
- Laboratory tests – routine haematology, biochemistry and urinalysis are beneficial in cases of sudden onset blindness because clinical signs and biochemical evidence of hyperadrenocorticism can occur in dogs with SARDS. Typical serum biochemical abnormalities in SARDS include elevated alkaline phosphatase (AP), alanine aminotransferase (ALT), cholesterol and bilirubin. Elevations in cortisol and sex hormones and proteinuria have also recently been shown in affected dogs (Carter *et al.*, 2009).

Although the serum biochemistry is abnormal in this dog (elevated AP, ALT, and cholesterol), the results of the ACTH-stimulation test and sex hormone levels are normal.

The remainder of the ophthalmic examination reveals no additional abnormalities and a general physical examination, including a neurological assessment, is unremarkable.

Diagnosis
Based on the information available, a diagnosis of SARDS is made.

Treatment
Currently, there is no treatment that can restore vision in dogs with SARDS. If there is concurrent hyperadrenocorticism, options to manage this disease should be discussed with the owners.

Intravenous therapy with human immunoglobulin (IVIg) has recently been described in a small number of dogs affected with SARDS and IMR with favourable results (Grozdanic *et al.*, 2008). IVIg has been used extensively in human medicine for a variety of immune-mediated diseases that are poorly responsive or non-responsive to traditional immunosuppressive therapy such as corticosteroids. The use of IVIg in dogs with SARDS and IMR is based on the belief that these conditions have features in common with antibody-mediated retinopathies in humans.

Prognosis

The prognosis for vision is hopeless in that the blindness caused by SARDS is permanent. In time, most affected dogs adapt and cope well. The systemic signs (polydipsia, polyuria, polyphagia) usually take several weeks to months to resolve unless hyperadrenocorticism is present, in which case specific treatment and long-term monitoring are indicated.

Discussion

The cause of SARDS is unknown. Although affected dogs may have concurrent hyperadrenocorticism, there is no evidence of an association with adrenal, pulmonary, or pituitary neoplasia, as there is in humans. An immune-mediated component has been postulated but studies looking for the presence of circulating retinal antibodies in affected dogs have so far produced contradictory findings. The initial abnormality involves the photoreceptor layer of the neurosensory retina, i.e. the rods and cones. On histopathology, the rod and cone photoreceptors initially undergo apoptosis, and degeneration of the remaining retina follows, resulting in end-stage retinal degeneration. The fundoscopic appearance several weeks to months after the onset of SARDS cannot be differentiated from generalised retinal degeneration resulting from other causes.

References and further reading

Carter RT, Oliver JW, Stepien RL, Bentley E (2009) Elevations in sex hormones in dogs with sudden acquired retinal degeneration syndrome (SARDS). *J Am Animal Hosp Assoc*, **45**, 207–214.

Grozdanic SD, Harper MH, Kecova H (2008) Antibody-mediated retinopathies in canine patients: mechanism, diagnosis, and treatment modalities. *Vet Clin North Am: Small Animal Pract*, **38** (2), 361–387.

See Appendix 2.

History

A 12-year-old female neutered domestic shorthaired cat is presented with a history of acute onset bilateral mydriasis and reduced vision five days after starting medication for a suspected tooth root abscess. The cat had lost weight over the previous few months but the owners assumed that this was because of its age. Based on an estimated bodyweight of 5 kg, the systemic medication consisted of enrofloxacin (an initial intravenous dose of 25 mg followed by 25 mg once daily *per os*, and oral meloxicam 1 mg/kg once daily).

Questions

1. Describe the abnormalities and pertinent normal features in Figs. 11.3a and b.
2. What differential diagnosis should be considered for this presentation?
3. What tests could you perform to make the diagnosis?

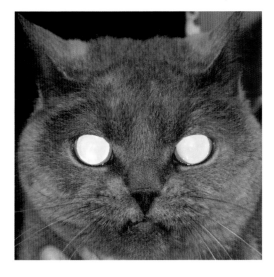

Fig. 11.3a

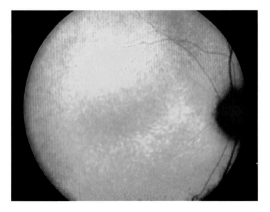

Fig. 11.3b Reproduced with permission from MM Ford.

Answers

1. What the figures show
Fig. 11.3a Both eyes – the pupil is very dilated.
Fig. 11.3b Right eye (tapetal fundus) – there is tapetal hyperreflectivity, which is predominantly central, and retinal vascular attenuation. Similar changes are present in the left eye (not shown).

2. Differential diagnoses
Given the history of sudden onset blindness together with bilateral retinal abnormalities, the following conditions should be considered:

- **Drug-associated retinal toxicity** The most significant ocular drug toxicity to be recently recognised in cats is enrofloxacin-associated retinal degeneration (Gelatt *et al.*, 2001; Ford *et al.*, 2007). Affected cats present with mydriasis and blindness which is usually permanent. Characteristic fundic abnormalities include tapetal hyperreflectivity, retinal vasculature attenuation, gold/rust-coloured spots in the tapetal fundus, and a pigmentary disturbance in the non-tapetal fundus. Other reported retinal toxins include the concurrent administration of methylnitrosourea and ketamine, and griseofulvin.
- **Retinitis/chorioretinitis** Active retinal inflammation (retinitis) typically appears as multiple areas of tapetal hyporeflectivity (dull, grey areas) sometimes with retinal haemorrhage. Post-inflammatory scarring is seen as areas of tapetal hyperreflectivity with or without pigment deposition and areas of depigmentation in the non-tapetal fundus. In the cat, chorioretinitis (choroidal inflammation that extends to the retina) is more common than retinochoroiditis (retinal inflammation that extends to the choroid). Causes of chorioretinitis in the cat include viral (e.g. feline infectious peritonitis virus), fungal (e.g. cryptococcosis), and protozoal infection (e.g. toxoplasmosis).
- **Retinal dysplasia** An abnormal development of the retina with proliferation of one or more of its elements. It is uncommon in the cat; however, retinal dysplasia has most often been associated with intrauterine or intraocular infection with FeLV. The typical fundoscopic appearance is multiple greyish dots or linear streaks which are most obvious in the tapetal fundus.
- **Nutritional retinal degeneration (taurine deficiency)** Taurine is an essential amino acid in the cat and the highest tissue concentrations are found in heart muscle, retina and liver. Fundic changes are bilaterally symmetrical – initially there is a focal area of tapetal hyperreflectivity dorsolateral to the optic disc and this ultimately progresses to generalised retinal degeneration (vascular attenuation and tapetal hyperreflectivity). Since the association between the dietary deficiency of taurine and the development of retinal disease was made in 1978, the condition has rarely been encountered, as dietary levels of taurine have been increased in commercial cat food.
- **Inherited rod-cone dysplasia and degeneration** Inherited retinal degeneration is rare in the cat. However, early-onset, autosomal recessive progressive retinal atrophy has been described in the Persian cat and affected cats are usually blind by four months of age (Rah *et al.*, 2005). The Abyssinian breed is known to be affected by two forms of inherited retinal degeneration, both of which have been described in detail. The first is an autosomal dominant rod-cone dysplasia that leads to blindness by one year of age; the second is an autosomal recessive rod-cone degeneration that leads to blindness by four to six years of age. The ophthalmoscopic appearance of these different forms of retinal degeneration is similar, i.e. tapetal hyperreflectivity, retinal vascular attenuation and depigmentation within the non-tapetal fundus.

3. Appropriate diagnostic tests
- Ocular reflexes
  - Pupillary light reflex – negative direct and consensual OU
  - Dazzle reflex – negative OU

- Vestibulo-oculocephalic reflex – positive OU
- Vision testing
  ◦ Menace response – negative OU
  ◦ Visual placing and tracking reflexes – negative OU
  ◦ Obstacle course – results are unreliable as the cat will not move around the consulting room.

In this cat, these finding are consistent with blindness in both eyes.

- Tonometry – IOP 20 mmHg OU

The bodyweight of the cat is 4.1 kg. The remainder of the ophthalmic examination and a general physical examination is unremarkable apart from dental disease.

Further diagnostic tests
- Electroretinography – this is not indicated because retinal function will be decreased if diffuse retinal degeneration is visible on fundoscopic examination.
- Laboratory tests – routine haematology, biochemistry, total T4 and urine analysis are unremarkable apart from mild azotaemia; urine specific gravity confirms adequate concentration consistent with dehydration.
- Systemic blood pressure measurement – indirect assessment with a Doppler sphygmomanometer (ultrasonic detection device) reveals an acceptable systolic blood pressure of 165 mmHg (upper limit for systolic blood pressure in the cat being 160–170 mmHg).

Diagnosis
Based on the information available, the cause of sudden blindness in this cat is presumed to be enrofloxacin-associated retinal degeneration.

Treatment
Immediate discontinuation of enrofloxacin therapy is indicated. Administration of intravenous fluid therapy has also been advocated, despite the fact that pharmacokinetics and metabolism of enrofloxacin are unknown in the cat. No other treatment options are available.

Prognosis
Blindness is usually permanent although there are reports of cats that have regained vision.

Discussion
A remarkable feature of enrofloxacin-associated toxicity is the speed at which the retina degenerates, and the fact that it can occur even after a single dose. The degeneration involves the outer layers of the retina, specifically the outer nuclear layer and the photoreceptors. Although all fluoroquinolones should be regarded as potentially retinotoxic at high doses, enrofloxacin in cats is the most relevant in the clinical setting.

Several important risk factors for enrofloxacin retinal toxicity have been identified (Wiebe et al., 2007). These include age (>12 years), pre-existing renal or hepatic impairment, dose and duration of treatment and route of administration. Retinotoxocity has been reported in cats even after treatment with the recommended dose, and for this reason enrofloxacin should only be used in cats when there is no alternative antibiotic therapy, i.e. its use should be based on culture and sensitivity testing. If treatment with enrofloxacin is necessary, the following guidelines should be closely adhered to: obtain an accurate bodyweight, do not exceed the recommended dose (5 mg/kg q24 hours), avoid intravenous administration, use a 1-ml syringe for accurate dosing (subcutaneous injection), assess renal and hepatic function by laboratory screening prior to drug administration, avoid in geriatric cats, and consider the effect of drug interactions, e.g. with systemic NSAID therapy. Age, undiagnosed systemic disease related to weight loss, inaccurate bodyweight, intravenous administration and concurrent NSAID therapy are identified as risk factors in this cat.

References and further reading

Ford MM, Dubielzig RR, Giuliano EA, Moore CP, Narfstrom KL (2007) Ocular and systemic manifestations after oral administration of a high dose of enrofloxacin in cats. *Am J Vet Res*, **68** (2), 190–202.

Gelatt KN, van der Woerdt A, Ketring KL, *et al.* (2001) Enrofloxacin-associated retinal degeneration in cats. *Vet Ophthalmol*, **4** (2), 99–106.

Rah H, Maggs DJ, Blankenship TN, *et al.* (2005) Early-onset, autosomal recessive, progressive retinal atrophy in Persian cats. *Invest Ophthalmol Visual Sci*, **46**, 1742–1747.

Wiebe V & Hamilton P (2002) Fluoroquinolone-induced retinal degeneration in cats. *J Am Vet Med Assoc*, **221**, 1568–1572.

See Appendix 2.

History

A 6-year-old male neutered terrier is presented with a history of occasionally bumping into objects on the left side over the past two to three days. During the same period, the owner has also noticed that the dog's eyes looked different from each other. The dog's general health had been unremarkable prior to the onset of this problem and he has received routine vaccinations and regular anthelmintic treatment. There is no travel history or changes in the dog's environment.

Questions

1. Describe the abnormalities and pertinent normal features in Figs. 11.4a and b.
2. What differential diagnoses should be considered for this presentation?
3. What tests could you perform to make the diagnosis?

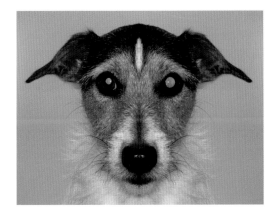

Fig. 11.4a

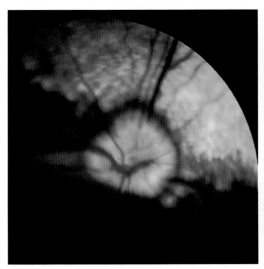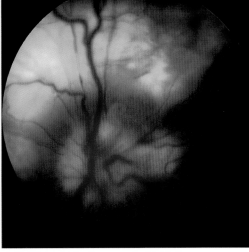

Fig. 11.4b

Answers

1. What the figures show

Fig. 11.4a Both eyes – there is a marked anisocoria (OS > OD); the blue tapetal reflection is a normal variation.

Fig. 11.4b Fundic photographs. Left eye – the optic disc is swollen and pink and has blurred indistinct margins. The blood vessels on and around the disc are engorged and tortuous, they appear to deviate from their normal path as they reach the disc. The peri-papillary region is hyporeflective, consistent with a retinal detachment. Right eye – the optic disc is normal. The irregular outline is because of pronounced myelination; the central grey area represents the physiological pit.

2. Differential diagnoses

Given the history and the appearance of the optic disc in the left eye, the following conditions should be considered:

- **Optic neuritis** Inflammation of the optic nerve can involve the intraocular (at the level of the optic disc), intraorbital (retrobulbar), or central portions of the nerve. Optic neuritis can be unilateral or bilateral and typically causes a sudden loss of vision and a reduced or absent PLR in the affected eye. The optic disc is swollen and raised; its margins may be blurred and haemorrhages may be present. However, if the intraocular portion of the nerve is unaffected, the fundus will appear normal. Electroretinography is expected to be normal with optic neuritis, as retinal function is generally unaffected. The following causes should be considered: idiopathic, inflammation, infection – viral (e.g. canine distemper virus, tick-borne encephalitis virus), fungal (e.g. *Blastomyces dermatitidis, Cryptococcosis neoformans, Histoplasma capsulatum*), bacterial (e.g. *Rickettsia rickettsii, Ehrlichia canis, Borrelia burgdorferii*), and protozoal (*Toxoplasma gondii, Neospora caninum*), neoplasia, granulomatous meningoencephalitis (GME or reticulosis), trauma and toxins (e.g. ivermectin). Optic neuritis is usually idiopathic in the dog.
- **Papilloedema** A non-inflammatory swelling of the optic disc usually associated with raised intracranial pressure, papilloedema is usually bilateral and, at least initially is not associated with visual or PLR deficits. Papilloedema has been reported in dogs with brain tumours; in contrast to humans, dogs rarely develop papilloedema secondary to raised intracranial pressure because they lack a central retinal artery and vein. Pseudo-papilloedema describes excessive myelination of the optic nerve axons beyond the anterior lamina cribosa, and is considered normal in the dog; it is seen in several breeds including the Golden Retriever and the German Shepherd Dog. Careful observation, and some experience is needed to differentiate papilloedema from pseudo-papilloedema, and therefore avoid unnecessary diagnostic procedures.
- **Optic nerve tumour** This is an uncommon tumour, but clinical signs include unilateral exophthalmos, mydriasis, papilloedema and/or optic neuritis. Clinical signs can arise as a result of primary tumours, e.g. optic nerve meningioma, nerve sheath tumour or secondary to local extension of orbital neoplasia.

3. Appropriate diagnostic tests

- Ocular reflexes
  - Pupillary light reflex – negative direct and consensual OS, positive direct and consensual OD
  - Dazzle reflex – negative OS, positive OD
  - Vestibulo-oculocephalic reflex – positive OU
- Vision testing
  - Menace response – negative OS, positive OD
  - Visual placing and tracking reflex – negative OS, positive OD

○ Obstacle course – the dog is unable to navigate around large objects in both photopic and scotopic conditions when the right eye is covered (patched); navigation is normal when the left eye is covered.

In this dog, these results are consistent with blindness in the left eye.

- Tonometry – IOP 19 mmHg OU

The remainder of the ophthalmic examination reveals no additional abnormalities and a general physical examination, including a neurological assessment, is unremarkable.

Further diagnostic tests

- Laboratory tests – routine haematology, biochemistry and urinalysis are indicated in cases of optic neuritis and papilloedema to screen for the presence of systemic disease; serology for infectious disease should be also considered, based on endemic diseases and travel history.

The results of routine haematology, biochemistry and urinalysis, and tests for *Toxoplasma gondii*, *Neospora caninum*, and *Ehrlichia canis* are normal in this dog.

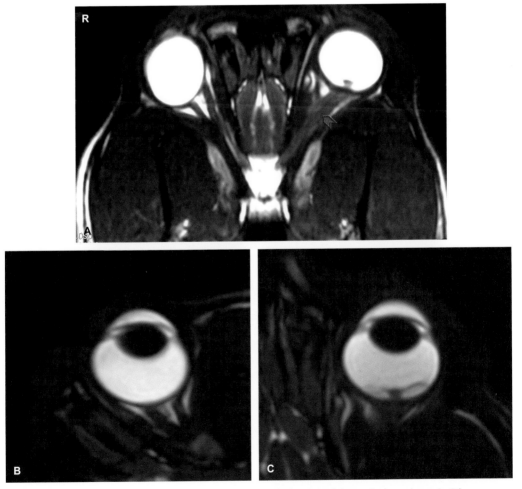

Fig. 11.4c MRI scans (dorsal plane 3D-fiesta). (A) Marked thickening of the optic nerve (arrow) with a swollen optic nerve head in the left eye. (B) Right eye – normal. (C) Left eye – swollen optic nerve head and peri-papillary retinal detachment.

- MRI scan – MRI is indicated to evaluate the retrobulbar portion of both optic nerves, the orbits and the brain in order to determine the extent and nature of the pathology. This has important implications for both treatment options and for prognosis.

  Abnormalities in the left eye include marked thickening of the optic nerve, a swollen optic nerve head and a peri-papillary retinal detachment (Fig. 11.4c). There is no evidence of orbital disease or brain involvement.

- Cerebrospinal fluid analysis – this is indicated to look for inflammation, infection or neoplasia. CSF analysis is normal.

Diagnosis

Based on the information available, a diagnosis of idiopathic optic neuritis in the left eye is made.

Treatment

Treatment for optic neuritis depends on the underlying cause. The treatment of choice for idiopathic optic neuritis is immunosuppressive doses of oral prednisolone, e.g. 4 mg/kg bodyweight per day for 48 hours, followed by 2 mg/kg per day until clinical signs resolve; the dose should then be tapered over two to three months. Early discontinuation of treatment carries the risk of recurrence. Close monitoring as the prednisolone is tapered is especially important in unilateral cases, as subtle changes in vision can easily be overlooked.

Prognosis and Discussion

The prognosis for return of vision with idiopathic optic neuritis is generally poor. Some eyes regain vision, often only temporarily, whilst others remain blind. Recurrence is possible and regular monitoring is indicated.

This dog does not respond to treatment and marked optic nerve atrophy develops within 10 days. Fundoscopic examination reveals a dark and small optic disc surrounded by pigmentation; the venous circle is barely visible because of attenuation of blood vessels (Fig. 11.4d).

Although optic neuritis may be unilateral, sudden onset blindness because of bilateral disease is the most common form in the dog. Both eyes may not be affected simultaneously, and the prognosis is generally better for the eye that is most recently affected.

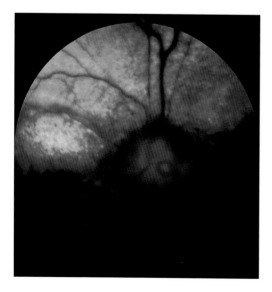

Fig. 11.4d Marked optic disc atrophy: a small and dark optic disc, attenuation of the venous circle and peri-papillary pigmentation.

References and further reading

Boroffka SA, Görig C, Auriemma E, Passon-Vastenburg MH, Voorhart G, Barthez PY (2008) MRI of the canine optic nerve. *Vet Radiol Ultrasound*, **49** (6), 540–544.

See Appendix 2.

History

An 8-year-old female neutered Collie-cross dog is presented with loss of vision over three to four days. The owner also reports that the dog appears depressed. The dog's general health has been unremarkable prior to the onset of this problem; she has received routine vaccinations and regular anthelmintic treatment.

Questions

1. Describe the abnormalities and pertinent normal features in Figs. 11.5a and b.
2. What differential diagnoses should be considered for this presentation?
3. What tests could you perform to make the diagnosis?

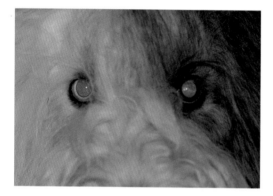

Fig. 11.5a Reproduced with permission from J Mould.

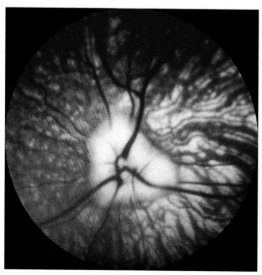
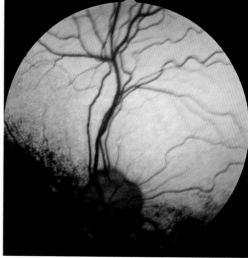

Fig. 11.5b

Answers

1. What the figures show
Fig. 11.5a Both eyes – the pupil is very dilated. The fundic reflection is a different colour in each eye – yellow in the left eye and red in the right eye. Both are normal variations in the dog. The red reflection is a result of subalbinism (reduced melanin in the hair and iris). The white coat and blue iris on the right side are also a result of subalbinism; the grey coat and brown iris on the left side indicate a normal level of melanin.

Fig. 11.5b Fundic photographs of the left and right eyes. Left eye – normal fundus with a yellow/green tapetal region; this results in the yellow fundic reflection seen in Fig. 11.5a. Right eye – subalbinotic fundus which is a normal variation in the dog. The choroidal vasculature (dense orange/red stripes) and sclera (white) can be directly observed because of the lack of melanin in the choroid and the overlying retinal pigmented epithelium, and the absence of a tapetum. The choroidal vasculature produces the red fundic reflection seen in Fig. 11.5a.

2. Differential diagnoses
Given the history and normal appearance of the fundus in both eyes, the following conditions should be considered for the cause of acute onset blindness:

- **Central blindness (amaurosis)** A lesion involving the central visual pathway can cause blindness. From the optic chiasm the optic tracts carry visual fibres which synapse within the lateral geniculate nucleus. Post-synaptic fibres then leave the lateral geniculate nucleus as the optic radiations, which terminate in the visual cortex of the cerebrum (lateral, causal and medial aspects of the occipital lobe).
- **Sudden acquired retinal degeneration syndrome (SARDS)** A retinal disorder of unknown cause that results in sudden onset blindness in affected dogs. The clinical presentation is characterised by a sudden loss of vision over several days to weeks which may be associated with polydipsia, polyuria, polyphagia and weight gain. Any breed or cross-breed dog can be affected and most affected animals are middle-aged. The fundus initially appears normal but signs of retinal degeneration (tapetal hyperreflectivity, retinal vascular attenuation and optic disc atrophy) develop over several months. Electroretinography produces a 'flat-line' response, consistent with a lack of retinal function (*case 2, this chapter*).
- **Optic neuritis** Inflammation of the optic nerve can affect the intraocular (at the level of the optic disc), intraorbital (retrobulbar) or central portion of the optic nerve. Optic neuritis can be unilateral or bilateral and typically causes a sudden loss of vision in the affected eye. The optic disc is swollen and raised; its margins may be blurred and haemorrhages may be present. However, if the intraocular portion of the nerve is unaffected, the fundus will appear normal. In contrast to SARDS, electroretinography is expected to be normal because retinal function is generally unaffected (*case 4, this chapter*).
- **Immune-mediated retinitis (IMR)** A syndrome recently described by veterinary ophthalmologists at Iowa State University. USA. The clinical appearance of dogs with IMR appears to be similar to that of SARDS. Investigations into the characterisation, diagnosis and treatment of this syndrome are on-going at the time of writing.

3. Appropriate diagnostic tests
- Ocular reflexes
  - Pupillary light reflex – negative direct and consensual OU
  - Dazzle reflex – negative OU
  - Vestibulo-oculocephalic reflex – positive OU

- Vision testing
  - Menace response – negative OU
  - Tracking reflex – negative OU
  - Obstacle course – the dog is unable to navigate around large objects under both photopic and scotopic conditions.

In this dog, these results suggest blindness in both eyes.

- Tonometry – IOP 20 mmHg OU

The remainder of the ophthalmic examination reveals no additional abnormalities and a general physical examination, including a neurological assessment, is unremarkable.

Further diagnostic tests

- Colourimetric pupillary light reflex testing – this is a recently described simple and inexpensive method for assessing photoreceptor and retinal ganglion cell function. This test investigates the response of the PLR to a red and blue light stimulus. If retinal function is reduced or absent and the disease involves the photoreceptor layer and/or the retinal ganglion cell layer, e.g. SARDS or IMR, the PLR is positive with a blue light stimulus but negative with a red light stimulus.

  In this dog, the direct and consensual PLR is negative with the standard white light as well as with the red and blue light stimuli. This is consistent with a disease process that does <u>not</u> involve the photoreceptor layer and/or the retinal ganglion cell layer.

- Laboratory tests – routine haematology, biochemistry and urine analysis are indicated if SARDS or optic neuritis is strongly suspected (*cases 2 and 4, this chapter*) and should also be considered prior to general anaesthesia in any middle-aged to older patient.

  In this dog, results of all laboratory tests are unremarkable.

- Electroretinography – this reveals b-wave amplitude and latency values which are considered to be within the normal range in both eyes, confirming the presence of satisfactory retinal function (Fig. 11.5c).

- MRI scan – electroretinography should ideally be performed prior to an MRI scan to rule out retinal causes of blindness first. This is because electroretinography is less expensive and can, in some dogs, be performed with sedation rather than under general anaesthesia (which is essential for MRI).

  An MRI scan to evaluate the optic nerve, orbit and brain in this dog reveals a lesion at the optic chiasm typical of a meningioma (Fig. 11.5d).

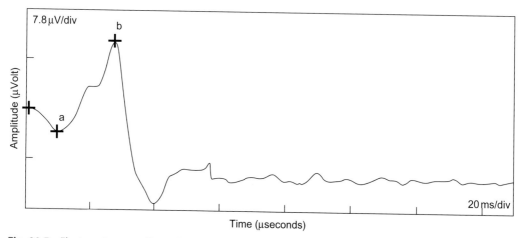

Fig. 11.5c Electroretinogram. Normal response confirms that satisfactory retinal function is present.

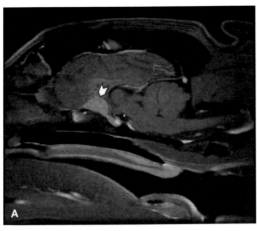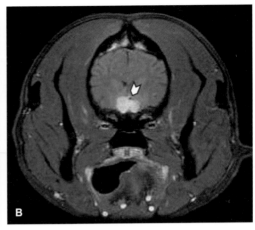

Fig. 11.5d MRI scans (T1 contrast images). (A) Sagittal scan. (B) Transverse scan. Meningioma at optic chiasm (arrow). Reproduced with permission from R Dennis, Animal Health Trust.

Diagnosis

Based on the information available, a diagnosis of central blindness (amaurosis) secondary to a meningioma involving the optic chiasm is made.

Treatment

Management options for intra-cranial meningiomas in the dog include corticosteroid therapy, radiotherapy and surgical excision. Systemic steroid therapy may be beneficial if there is oedema surrounding the tumour, as it can temporarily improve demeanour and lead to return of vision in some dogs. Optic chiasm meningiomas in the dog are suitable for radiotherapy. Surgery is not an option for the meningioma in this dog because of its location. A detailed discussion of the treatment options for meningioma is beyond the scope of this book.

Prognosis

The prognosis for survival of a dog with an intra-cranial meningioma is poor. The median survival for a brain meningioma in dogs treated with systemic corticosteroid therapy only is 58 days; this can be increased to seven to nine months with tumour resection or radiotherapy. The best long-term median survival is 16.5 months with a combination of tumour resection (when possible) and radiotherapy (Axlund *et al.*, 2002).

Discussion

Both pituitary gland tumours and meningiomas can involve the optic chiasm and cause blindness. Most pituitary gland tumours expand dorsally into the hypothalamus (away from the optic chiasm) and tend not to cause visual impairment until the tumour is relatively advanced.

Other causes of central blindness include congenital (e.g. hydrocephalus), inflammatory (e.g. granulomatous meningoencephalitis), metabolic (e.g. hepatic encephalopathy), infectious (e.g. canine distemper virus), vascular disease (e.g. infarction), and trauma. With central blindness, concurrent systemic or neurologic signs are often present and require further investigation. Advanced imaging techniques (MRI and CT) are essential for accurate diagnosis and prognosis and for the consideration of management and treatment options in animals with suspected central blindness.

References and further reading

Axlund TW, McGlasson ML, Smith AN (2002) Surgery alone or in combination with radiation therapy for treatment of intracranial meningiomas in dogs: 31 cases (1989–2002). *J Am Vet Med Assoc*, **221**(11), 1597–1600.

Grozdanic SD, Harper MH, Kecova H (2008) Antibody-mediated retinopathies in canine patients: mechanism, diagnosis, and treatment modalities. *Vet Clin North Am: Small Animal Pract*, **38** (2), 361–387.

See Appendix 2.

CHAPTER 12

Ocular Trauma

Introduction

Most ocular trauma involves loss of vision, compromised globe integrity or severe ocular pain. The majority of ocular emergencies are traumatic in origin, and prompt action is required, as delay in treating may result in a blind eye or necessitate enucleation. Following trauma the appearance of the eye is often dramatic and animals are reluctant to allow thorough evaluation; the eye may be partially closed, making assessment of the ocular reflexes particularly difficult to interpret. Observation from a distance first is usually helpful, but it may be necessary to sedate an animal before a thorough examination can be performed; if sedation is required it is essential to assess the general condition of the animal first.

Small Animal Ophthalmology: What's Your Diagnosis? First Edition. Heidi Featherstone, Elaine Holt.
© 2011 by Heidi Featherstone and Elaine Holt. Published 2011 by Blackwell Publishing Ltd.

History

A two-year-old male neutered Lhasa Apso is presented 10 days after treatment for proptosis of the left eye following a dog fight. Emergency treatment had consisted of repositioning the eye under general anaesthesia, a temporary tarsorrhaphy and systemic broad-spectrum antibiotic and NSAID therapy. The tarsorrhapy sutures are removed to allow examination of the eye.

Questions

1. Describe the abnormalities and pertinent normal features in Figs. 12.1a and b.
2. What differential diagnoses should be considered for this presentation?
3. What tests could you perform to make the diagnosis?

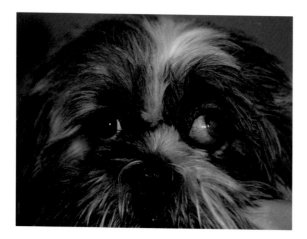

Fig. 12.1a

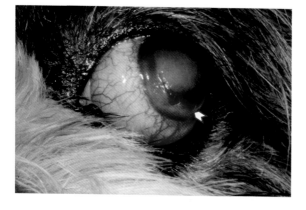

Fig. 12.1b

Answers

1. What the figures show

Fig. 12.1a The right eye appears normal. Left eye – there is a marked lateral deviation of the eye (lateral strabismus or exotropia) resulting in increased exposure of the medial region of the bulbar conjunctiva and sclera and a wide palpebral fissure (OS > OD). There is conjunctival hyperaemia, a generalised corneal opacity and the Purkinje images are disrupted.

Fig. 12.1b Left eye – there is diffuse oedema and peri-limbal corneal vascularisation. The blood vessels in the conjunctiva and the episclera are hyperaemic and there is an irregular line of grey tissue which represents the outline of a superficial ulcer (arrow). The upper and lower eyelids and TEL are in a normal position.

2. Differential diagnoses

Given the history and the appearance of the left eye, it is possible to make an immediate diagnosis of exotropia and keratitis secondary to traumatic proptosis of the left eye. It is, however, important to distinguish between proptosis and exophthalmos:

- **Proptosis** Proptosis results from the sudden forward displacement of the eye with simultaneous entrapment and inversion of the eyelids behind the equator of the eye. Entrapment prevents the eye from spontaneously returning to its normal position, an effect exacerbated by orbital soft tissue swelling resulting from impaired venous drainage (Fig. 12.1c). Proptosis is the result of trauma, and brachycephalic breeds are predisposed because of their shallow orbits. To a veterinary surgeon not experienced with this condition, there may be concern in this dog that the globe is still displaced from its normal position within the orbit.

- **Exophthalmos** (*Ch. 1, case 3*) Exophthalmos can exist following replacement of a proptosed globe because of soft tissue swelling and the formation of a haematoma in the retrobulbar space. Fractures and emphysema (from a fracture involving the frontal sinus) can also contribute to exophthalmos. Orbital fractures are usually sustained from severe blunt trauma, e.g. a kick by a horse, and are less likely to arise from a dog fight unless there is a considerable difference in size between the dogs involved. Unlike proptosis, the eyelid margins are not inverted with exophthalmos.

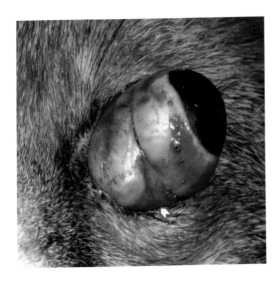

Fig. 12.1c Proptosis of the left eye of a young, mixed-breed dog following a road traffic accident. Note the position of the eyelid margins which are inverted and positioned behind the equator of the globe (arrow).

3. Appropriate diagnostic tests

- Ocular reflexes
  - Pupillary light reflex – corneal oedema prevents observation of the pupil in the left eye. Negative consensual OS (left to right eye), positive direct OD.
  - Dazzle reflex – negative OS, positive OD
  - Palpebral reflex – negative OS, positive but incomplete OD; the incomplete palpebral reflex in the right eye is consistent with breed-related lagophthalmos (*Ch.8, case 3*).
  - Corneal reflex – negative OS, positive OD (Fig. 12.1d)

Corneal sensation can be assessed by touching a wisp of cotton wool to the lateral region of the cornea, i.e. away from the visual axis; if a blink response is elicited, corneal sensation is said to be present (*Ch.8, case 4*). In an eye with marked surface pathology, a cotton bud can also be used; in a blind eye the stimulus can be applied to any part of the cornea (Fig. 12.1d).

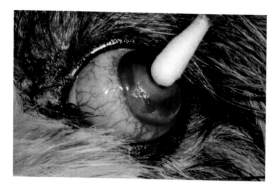

Fig. 12.1d Left eye following application of fluorescein dye. Positive fluorescein retention reveals a large superficial corneal ulcer.

- Menace response – negative OS, positive OD

In this dog, these results are consistent with loss of vision, and loss of corneal and eyelid sensation in the left eye.

- Examination with a focal light source – in the left eye, slit-lamp biomicroscopy determines that the corneal vascularisation is both superficial and deep, and that the corneal thickness is increased.
- Schirmer tear test – 5 mm/min OS, 17 mm/min OD. Given the overall clinical presentation, the low tear production in the left eye is most consistent with reduced reflex tear production because of the loss of corneal sensation, as well as possible damage to the lacrimal and TEL glands.
- Fluorescein dye – large superficial area of positive staining OS, negative OD (Fig. 12.1e)
- Tonometry – IOP 18 mmHg OS, 15 mmHg OD

The remainder of the ophthalmic examination reveals no additional abnormalities and a general physical examination is unremarkable.

Diagnosis

Based on the results of the ophthalmic examination, a more specific diagnosis of blindness and neurotrophic keratitis in the left eye is made. The blindness is considered to be irreversible because the trauma to the optic nerve occurred 10 days ago.

Treatment

Enucleation is recommended in this dog because of irreversible blindness and loss of corneal sensation in the left eye. Enucleation of a blind and comfortable eye following traumatic proptosis is not

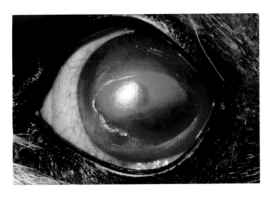

Fig. 12.1e Left eye following application of fluorescein dye. Positive fluorescein retention reveals a large superficial corneal ulcer.

always necessary. However, concurrent corneal desensitisation leads to neurotrophic keratitis which can in turn give rise to complications (chronic corneal ulceration, corneal neovascularisation, secondary bacterial infection and ultimately corneal perforation) which necessitate removal.

The eye is removed by a routine transconjunctival procedure and submitted for histopathology. Postoperative treatment comprises systemic broad-spectrum antibiotic and NSAID therapy for five days.

Histopathological examination confirms chronic ulcerative keratitis and reveals severe degeneration and atrophy of the optic nerve – the latter consistent with tractional injury secondary to proptosis.

> All enucleated globes should be submitted for ocular histopathology. For routine diagnostic purposes, fixation of the globe in 10% formalin is generally appropriate, although confirmation with the selected laboratory is recommended. Prior to fixation, as much excess extraocular tissue as possible should be removed, and the optic nerve should be left as long as possible.

Prognosis and Discussion

It is important to try to determine the prognosis for vision and for the eye itself when considering the treatment plan for a proptosed eye. The prognosis for vision is poor, as only about 20% of eyes retain vision following traumatic proptosis, although prognosis is influenced by the breed of dog. Relatively little force is required to proptose the eye in brachycephalic breeds compared to dolichocephalic breeds. Fortunately proptosis occurs more frequently in brachycephalic breeds for which the prognosis for vision is generally more favourable. However, the prognosis for each dog should be assessed on an individual basis based on the following guidelines:

- Reasons for immediate enucleation
  - Avulsion of the optic nerve (usually apparent on examination)
  - Corneal or scleral rupture, indicated by loss of the normal shape and turgidity of the eye
  - Extensive damage to the extraocular muscles – this can result in irreversible compromise of the vascular and nerve supply to the anterior segment of the eye, and the development of neurotrophic keratitis
- Positive prognostic indicators
  - Presence of a direct and consensual pupillary light reflex and/or evidence of vision at initial presentation
  - Mild degree of proptosis
  - Damage to more than three extraocular muscles
  - Absent or minor intraocular haemorrhage

- Pupil size is variable and is not considered to be a useful prognostic indicator by many ophthalmologists
- An eye with extensive intraocular haemorrhage has a guarded prognosis but can be surgically replaced and enucleated later if necessary.

In reality, accurate assessment of the degree of damage to the extraocular muscles can be difficult and common sense prevails. The medial, ventral and ventral oblique recti are the shortest extraocular muscles and usually rupture first. This results in exotropia which is a common clinical sign at the time of the injury and following replacement of the eye. Surgical reattachment of the torn muscles is usually impractical and is rarely performed. Exotropia will improve and can even resolve with time.

Poor ocular surface health is a common long-term problem following replacement of a proptosed eye. Ocular surface disease should be managed with topical lubricant therapy and/or surgically with a bilateral medial canthoplasty. The benefits of a medial canthoplasty include improved blinking, reduced exposure of the ocular surface, coverage of the exposed medial aspect in an eye with exotropia and a reduced risk of repeat globe prolapse.

The long-term sequelae of globe proptosis include blindness, lateral strabismus (exotropia), lagophthalmos, exposure keratitis, keratoconjunctivitis sicca, neurotrophic keratitis, glaucoma and phthisis bulbi. Although most owners prefer a blind, comfortable eye to enucleation, many will not wish to provide frequent medical care for a blind eye indefinitely. If there is any doubt whether the eye can be salvaged, it is acceptable to replace the eye as an emergency procedure and then, if necessary, to enucleate it later.

Further reading
See Appendix 2.

History

A three-year-old female neutered domestic shorthaired cat is presented with evidence of acute trauma to the left eye; the cat is subdued and reluctant to move. She has received routine vaccinations and anthelmintic treatment and is an indoor/outdoor cat.

Questions

1. Describe the abnormalities and pertinent normal features in Fig. 12.2a.
2. What differential diagnoses should be considered for this presentation?
3. What tests could you perform to make the diagnosis?

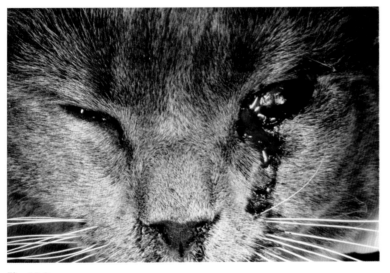

Fig. 12.2a

Answers

1. What the figure shows
Fig. 12.2a There is dried blood on the left side of the face and around both nostrils. Left eye – there is blood at the medial canthus. The palpebral fissure is wide (OS > OD). The ocular surface has a lack-lustre appearance and is a red/black colour – intraocular structures are not visible through this dark opaque surface. The Purkinje images are disrupted. Right eye – is virtually closed and the Purkinje images are normal.

2. Differential diagnoses
Given the appearance of the left eye, the following conditions should be considered:

- **Globe rupture** This can result from penetrating or blunt trauma. Penetrating trauma can involve the cornea and/or sclera, although the cornea is more likely to be involved because of its exposed position. Corneal lacerations can extend across the limbus into the sclera and may be obscured by conjunctival chemosis and haemorrhage. In dogs and cats, scleral rupture usually results from blunt trauma and is often located at the posterior pole, sometimes at the equator. Scleral rupture is associated with acute pain and mild to extensive intraocular haemorrhage. The loss of aqueous or vitreous humour secondary to corneal laceration or scleral rupture results in reduced globe turgidity. There may be concurrent damage to the lens (e.g. luxation and/or rupture), uveal tract (e.g. avulsion) or orbital tissues (e.g. haematoma, emphysema and fractures).
- **Intraocular haemorrhage** Causes include trauma, uveitis, chronic glaucoma, neoplasia (primary or secondary), pre-iridal fibrovascular membranes, systemic disease (e.g. hypertension, coagulopathy and platelet disorders) and, rarely, congenital anomalies (e.g. persistent hyaloid artery, persistent hyperplastic primary vitreous) (*Ch. 1, case 1*).
- **Proptosis** This results from the sudden forward displacement of the eye with simultaneous entrapment and inversion of the eyelids behind the equator of the eye. The eyelid entrapment prevents the eye from spontaneously returning to its normal position, and this effect is exacerbated by orbital soft tissue swelling because of impaired venous drainage (*case 1, this chapter*). The feline orbit provides better protection for the eye than the canine orbit, which means that considerable force is required to cause proptosis in the cat and concurrent head trauma is often present.

3. Appropriate diagnostic tests
The eye is too painful for a complete ophthalmic examination; a limited examination is performed:

- Pupillary light reflex – the pupil in the left eye is not visible; negative consensual OS, positive direct OD.
- Dazzle reflex – negative OS, positive OD

No abnormalities are found in the right eye. The physical examination is unremarkable apart from dried blood at both nares. Given that the cat appears stable, it is anaesthetised to allow closer examination of the eye and periocular area. Once the periocular hair is clipped and the ocular surface flushed, the following abnormalities are revealed: eyelid bruising, subconjunctival haemorrhage, and a full thickness wound in the lower eyelid (Fig. 12.2b). The globe appears to be intact – this is determined by the impression of a formed rather than collapsed globe.

The following diagnostic tests are performed to evaluate the nature of the injury in the left eye in more detail:

- B-mode ocular ultrasound – this is performed on both eyes for comparison. The right eye is unremarkable. In the left eye there is a deep anterior chamber (9 mm as compared to 3.5 mm

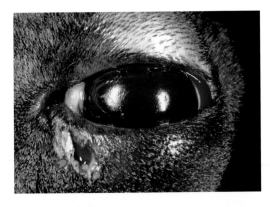

Fig. 12.2b Full thickness skin wound later identified as entry point for airgun pellet (arrow).

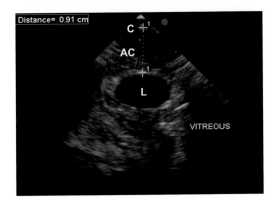

Fig. 12.2c B-mode ultrasound scan. Left eye – deep anterior chamber, posterior displacement of the lens and no visible outline for the posterior wall of the globe. AC, anterior chamber; C, cornea; L, lens.

OD), hyperechoic material in the anterior chamber and the vitreous cavity, and no visible posterior outline of the globe. These findings are consistent with posterior displacement of the lens, intraocular haemorrhage and posterior scleral rupture (Fig. 12.2c).

- Radiography – skull radiography reveals a metallic foreign body consistent with an airgun pellet. The pellet is dorsal to the soft palate and rostral to the left tympanic bulla (Fig. 12.2d).

Diagnosis
Based on the information available, a diagnosis of a traumatic posterior scleral rupture of the left eye is made.

Treatment
Posterior scleral rupture often results in catastrophic damage to intraocular structures and is usually permanently blinding. Affected eyes are painful and there is a long-term risk of the development of feline post-traumatic ocular sarcoma (see Discussion below). Enucleation is frequently the only sensible course of action.

The eye is removed by a routine transconjunctival procedure; gross examination confirms a posterior lens luxation and a focal posterior scleral rupture (Fig. 12.2e).

Prognosis
The prognosis for a full recovery following enucleation is excellent in this cat. Airgun pellets are inert and rarely require removal if they remain in a clinically insignificant location such as in this cat.

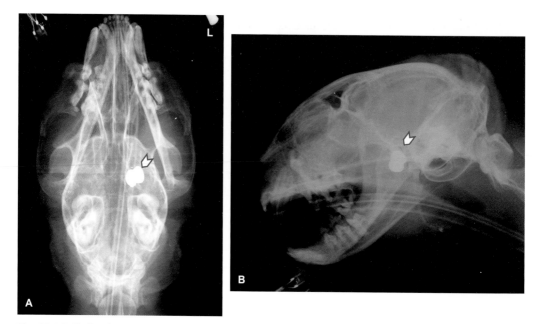

Fig. 12.2d Skull radiographs. (A) Dorsoventral view. (B) Lateral view. An airgun pellet (arrow) is located at the base of the skull, dorsal to the hard palate and rostral to the left tympanic bulla.

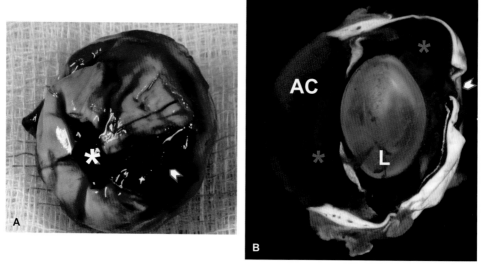

Fig. 12.2e (A) Enucleated globe showing posterior scleral rupture (arrow) and position of the optic nerve (asterix). (B) Gross pathology showing deep anterior chamber, intraocular haemorrhage (asterix), posterior displacement of the lens and scleral rupture (arrow). AC, anterior chamber; L, lens. Reproduced with permission from EJ Scurrell.

Discussion

Traumatic posterior scleral ruptures are common in cats and dogs. The injury is usually the result of blunt trauma but can also result from direct penetration of the globe. Accidental scleral rupture is also known to occur during dental procedures. The floor of the orbit in carnivores consists of soft tissue rather than bone and the distance between the upper dental arcade and the eye is small – both these factors increase the risk of accidental scleral laceration by dental instruments. Lacerations or ruptures involving the cornea or the anterior region of the sclera are usually easily identified, whereas a posterior scleral rupture can be difficult to diagnose even with the aid of ultrasound. In a retrospective study in dogs, cats and horses, scleral rupture was only diagnosed prior to enucleation in 2 out of 30 affected eyes; the most common site for rupture was the posterior pole around the optic nerve, and the most frequent clinical signs were eyelid and conjunctival swelling, subconjunctival haemorrhage and hyphaema (Rampazzo et al., 2006). In the authors' experience, eyes with posterior scleral ruptures are soft or sunken and very painful on palpation. It is, however, possible for the shape and size of the eye to appear normal initially, as orbital haemorrhage can effectively seal the site of the rupture. Mild exophthalmos sometimes results from orbital haemorrhage and soft tissue swelling. If enucleation is not performed, the extensive damage to intraocular structures causes eventual atrophy of the globe (phthisis bulbi).

One important reason to consider enucleation of a traumatised eye, specifically in the cat, is the potential for the development of a feline post-traumatic ocular sarcoma. This is an uncommon but highly malignant neoplasm which is usually associated with a previous history of ocular trauma and lens injury. Affected cats range from 7 to 15 years and the interval between the traumatic event and the detection of the tumour averages five years. The clinical presentation is unilateral and can include signs of chronic uveitis, glaucoma, intraocular haemorrhage and a white/pink mass in the posterior segment. The prognosis is poor following enucleation or exenteration as the majority of cats die from the effects of local extension and/or metastatic disease within several months. In the dog it may be acceptable to maintain a blind but comfortable eye following trauma (*Ch. 12, case 1*) as there are no known risks of trauma-induced neoplasia.

References and further reading

Rampazzo A, Eule C, Speier S, Grest P, Spiess B (2006) Scleral rupture in dogs, cats and horses. *Vet Ophthalmol*, **9** (3), 149–155.

See Appendix 2.

History

A three-year-old male Papillon is presented with bleeding from the left eye after being attacked by a cat. The dog has received routine vaccinations and anthelmintic treatment and is otherwise well.

Questions

1. Describe the abnormalities and pertinent normal features in Figs. 12.3a and b.
2. What differential diagnoses should be considered for this presentation?
3. What tests could you perform to make the diagnosis?

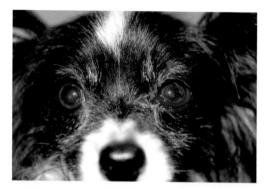

Fig. 12.3a

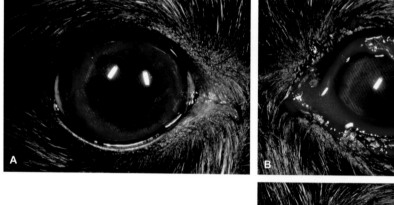

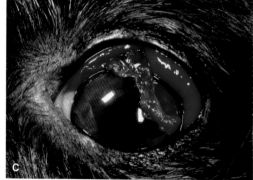

Fig. 12.3b (A) Right eye (B) Left eye at presentation (C) Left eye after the haemorrhage has been removed.

Answers

1. What the figures show
Fig. 12.3 The right eye appears normal. Left eye – there is haemorrhage on the ocular surface which appears recent. The eye appears smaller than the right and the pupil is miotic, resulting in a relative anisocoria (OS < OD).

Fig. 12.3b Left eye – a ragged piece of conjunctival tissue lies over the dorsal region of the cornea. There is considerable swelling of the dorsal bulbar conjunctiva and subconjunctival haemorrhage. The Purkinje images are normal.

2. Differential diagnoses
Given the history and the appearance of the left eye, the clinical diagnosis is ocular haemorrhage secondary to trauma. The location and extent of the trauma is important to consider so that appropriate decisions can be made with regard to treatment.

- **Extraocular trauma** Sharp trauma can cause partial thickness lacerations to the conjunctiva and cornea; the cornea is often involved because of its exposed position. Corneal lacerations can extend across the limbus into the sclera but limbal/scleral involvement may be obscured by conjunctival chemosis and haemorrhage. With partial thickness injuries, the pupil size can be miotic because of reflex uveitis but it should be a normal shape; dyscoria will only occur from penetrating trauma involving the iris.
- **Intraocular trauma** A full thickness injury is usually restricted to the anterior segment but can involve the posterior segment. As with extraocular trauma, the pupil may be miotic because of reflex uveitis but dyscoria is common and provides supportive evidence for a penetrating injury involving the iris. Intraocular haemorrhage is also common and may be restricted to the anterior chamber (hyphaema) and/or involve the vitreous humour – blood in the vitreous humour appears as a red haze behind the pupil. Careful examination for signs of lens trauma is important, as lens involvement will affect both treatment and prognosis. Observation of the lens is often restricted by concurrent miosis and dilation of the pupil is required for a thorough assessment – injury to the lens usually appears as a white opacity which is visible through the pupil. The nature of the ocular discharge can provide additional information about the location of the injury. A serous discharge occurs with increased lacrimation and escape of aqueous humour; a gelatinous discharge is produced by coagulated aqueous humour or prolapsed vitreous humour.

3. Appropriate diagnostic tests
- Ocular reflexes
  - Pupillary light reflex – direct and consensual positive OU
  - Dazzle reflex – positive OU
  - Palpebral reflex – positive OU
- Menace response – positive OU
- Examination with a focal light source – the right eye appears normal. The depth and transparency of the anterior chamber is normal in the left eye. Examination of the left eye for a corneal or conjunctival foreign body is facilitated by the use of topical anaesthesia – no foreign body is found. Both topical 0.5% tropicamide and 0.5% atropine eye drops are administered to dilate the pupil. (Atropine is used because it is a more potent mydriatic/cycloplegic drug and the miosis in the left eye is likely to be a manifestation of anterior uveitis. The administration of both drugs may help to save time rather than waiting for the effect of tropicamide alone because it may not be potent enough to cause mydriasis.) Intraocular examination is repeated – no intraocular

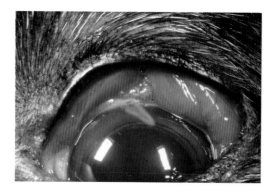

Fig. 12.3c Left eye following application of fluorescein dye. A superficial laceration in the dorsal peripheral cornea appears as an area of positive linear fluorescein retention.

abnormalities are observed. Mild haemorrhage continues intermittently throughout the examination and its precise origin cannot be determined at this stage.

- Schirmer tear test – this is not performed in the left eye because of the haemorrhage. It is also not performed in the right eye to minimise stress to the dog and because of the appearance of a good tear film.
- Fluorescein dye
  - Staining – negative OD, linear positive staining in the dorsal peripheral cornea OS. This is consistent with a superficial corneal laceration in the left eye (Fig. 12.3c).
  - Seidel test – negative OU
- Tonometry – IOP 12 mmHg OS, 15 mmHg OD

The remainder of the examination of the right eye, and a general physical examination, are unremarkable.

Tropicamide is a parasympatholytic agent that causes mydriasis but not cycloplegia. It a useful drug to dilate the pupil for an ophthalmic examination because it has a relatively rapid onset (20–30 min) and a relatively short duration of action (4–6 h). Atropine is a parasympatholytic agent with potent mydriatic and cycloplegic effects. It has a relatively slow onset of action (about 1 h) and a long duration of action (up to 5 days in the dog and 2–3 days in the cat), and it is used therapeutically for uveitis.

Diagnosis

Based on the information available, the findings are consistent with conjunctival and corneal trauma to the left eye.

Treatment

Examination under general anaesthesia is important for two reasons – firstly, to identify the origin of the haemorrhage and secondly, to explore the conjunctival wound in order to eliminate the presence of scleral involvement. The piece of torn conjunctiva is excised and exploration of the area reveals the source of the haemorrhage to be a scleral blood vessel which is several millimetres posterior to the limbus – diathermy is applied to control the haemorrhage (Fig. 12.3d). The injuries to the cornea, conjunctiva and sclera are superficial and are left to heal by second intention.

Topical atropine (0.5%) is applied 'to effect' to dilate the pupil and relieve iridociliary muscle spasm, i.e. q12 h for two days, then q24 h for two days and then q3 days on two occasions. Topical

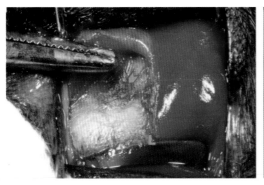

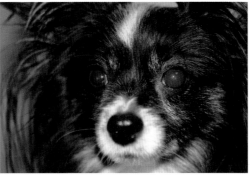

Fig. 12.3d Dorsal bulbar conjunctiva has been incised and reflected to show a focal brown area on the surface of the sclera (arrow) which represents the site of diathermy application. L, limbus.

Fig. 12.3e Ten days after treatment – the left pupil is dilated from topical atropine.

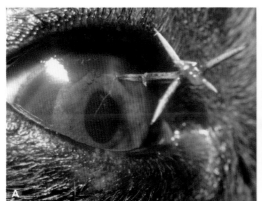

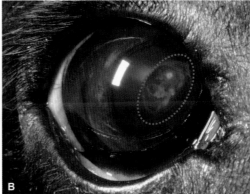

Fig. 12.3f (A) Thorn injury in a dog. (B) Traumatic cataract (blue circle) following a penetrating injury from a cat scratch in a Labrador puppy, visible only after the pupil was dilated.

and systemic Broad-spectrum antibiotic and systemic NSAID therapy are also prescribed for seven days.

Prognosis

The prognosis for a full recovery is considered excellent in this dog (Fig. 12.3e).

Discussion

Penetrating ocular trauma is common in dogs and cats, particularly from thorn and cat scratch injuries (Fig. 12.3f). A thorough examination, often under sedation/anaesthesia, is indicated to determine the full extent of the injury. It is not uncommon for small penetrating corneal injuries to seal (i.e. not stain with fluorescein) rapidly, even within 24 hours. This can mask a more serious problem involving the intraocular structures. An injury to the lens is particularly serious and can easily be missed if the pupil is not dilated for examination. A short-acting mydriatic agent such as tropicamide may not be sufficiently potent to induce mydriasis in an eye with anterior uveitis from trauma, and a more potent mydriatic and cycloplegic agent such as atropine should be considered.

Small tears in the anterior lens capsule can heal spontaneously but large tears and traumatic cataract formation should be managed surgically by early lens extraction (phacoemulsification) (*Ch. 7, case 2*). If a full thickness penetrating injury with significant associated lens trauma is overlooked and left untreated, the resulting phacoclastic uveitis and secondary glaucoma will necessitate enucleation.

Further reading
See Appendix 2.

Practical Tips for An Ophthalmic Examination

A thorough and systematic ophthalmic examination is essential to reach a diagnosis. Most veterinary ophthalmology textbooks (see Appendix 2) provide detailed descriptions of how to perform an ophthalmic examination.

The purpose of this appendix is to explain and clarify those aspects of the ophthalmic examination which are used in this book. They provide helpful clinical information and are widely used by clinical ophthalmologists. This section also provides the reference ranges for the standard ophthalmic diagnostic tests used in the book.

Pupillary light reflex (PLR)

(i) Direct PLR
Constriction of the pupil when a light is shone in the eye.

(ii) Consensual or indirect PLR
Constriction of the pupil when a light is shone in the opposite eye (for example, a positive consensual PLR in the left eye means the right pupil constricts when a light is shone in the left eye). That is the definition used in this book. Note that some authors use the term the other way around (a positive consensual PLR in the left eye would mean the left pupil constricting when a light is shone in the right eye).

Examination with a focal light source
A focal rather than diffuse light source is preferred for the ophthalmic examination. It helps in the general examination of the anterior segment (cornea, anterior chamber, iris, lens) and adnexa, and is also used to elicit basic ocular reflexes, such as the PLR and dazzle reflex. An otoscope (with speculum removed) and a Finnoff transilluminator are good examples of focal light sources, whereas a pen torch has a relatively diffuse beam. The direct ophthalmoscope is not appropriate for assessing the PLR because it provides low light intensity; the instrument is designed for viewing the fundus with minimal constriction of the pupil. Indeed, it can create false-negative results for the PLR and dazzle reflex because of its low light intensity.

Purkinje images (or Purkinje-Sanson images)
These are formed by light reflecting from the outer cornea (precorneal tear film and anterior corneal surface), inner cornea, anterior lens and posterior lens. The effect is shown clearly in photographs

Small Animal Ophthalmology: What's Your Diagnosis? First Edition. Heidi Featherstone, Elaine Holt.
© 2011 by Heidi Featherstone and Elaine Holt. Published 2011 by Blackwell Publishing Ltd.

with the reflection of the camera flash. The Purkinje image caused by reflection of light on the outer cornea is the most helpful clinically. If the ocular surface is smooth, the outline of the image is sharply defined and the shape of the image corresponds to the shape of the light source (Fig. 5.2c, E). Assessment of the Purkinje images provides information about the nature of the precorneal tear film and the regularity of the corneal surface. If the anterior corneal surface is diseased, e.g. corneal ulcer, the Purkinje images are also disrupted (Figs 5.2c, A). If the precorneal tear film is deficient, e.g. in an eye with keratoconjunctivitis sicca, the Purkinje images are disrupted (Fig. 4.3b).

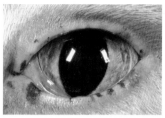
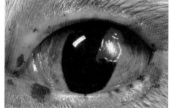
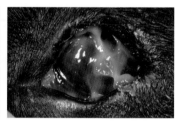

Fig. 5.2c, E   **Fig. 5.2c, A**   **Fig. 4.3b**

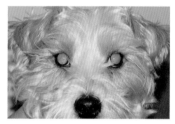
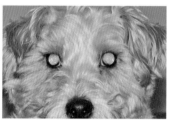
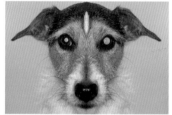

Fig. 7.1a Adult terrier with mature cataract in both eyes. The pupils appear white (leukocoria) and the tapetal reflection is absent in both eyes. Reproduced with permission from J Mould.

Fig. 7.1f Adult terrier following bilateral cataract surgery and placement of artificial intraocular lenses. The tapetal reflection is restored in both eyes. Reproduced with permission from J Mould.

Fig. 11.4a Adult terrier with anisocoria.

Tapetal reflection (or tapetal reflex, fundic reflex)

This is the reflection of light from the tapetal fundus through the pupil, best seen at a distance. Tapetal reflection is the reason for 'eye shine' when animals are illuminated in car headlights at night. Humans do not have a tapetum but still demonstrate a fundic reflex, seen as 'red eye' in photographs. For a normal tapetal reflection the visual axis must be clear, i.e. the path from the tapetum (in the choroid) through the retina, vitreous humour, lens, aqueous humour, cornea to the precorneal tear film (Fig. 11.3a). Any opacity in the pathway will obstruct the passage of light and cause an abnormal tapetal reflection, e.g. cataract, iris cyst. A mature cataract is the opacity of the entire lens – it will block the tapetal reflection completely (Figs 7.1a, c, and f). An iris cyst causes only a focal opacity in the tapetal reflection (Fig. 9.1e). Tapetal reflection can also help to determine if there is a size difference between the pupils, i.e. anisocoria (Fig. 11.4a). The colour of the tapetum varies between species and between individual animals (Figs 10.2b, and 11.5a).

Dazzle reflex

When a *bright* focal light source is shone in the eye, the normal response is a bilateral, partial eyelid blink. The anatomical pathway for the dazzle reflex has not been elucidated in animals but evidence from human literature suggests that it is present when the optic nerve is intact to the level of the midbrain, most likely the area of the rostral colliculus. The retina and optic nerve (cranial nerve II), the facial nerve (cranial nerve VII) and the orbicularis oculi muscle form an integral part of this reflex. The dazzle reflex is a subcortical reflex and suggests that there is the ability to detect a *bright* light.

Tear film break-up time (TBUT)

This is a measure of the stability of the tear film and is used in the diagnosis of qualitative tear film disorders. It involves measuring the time it takes for the tear film to dissociate from the ocular surface. Fluorescein dye is applied to the ocular surface; the eye is allowed to blink, then the eyelids are held open and the time until the first dark spot in the fluorescein appears is measured. Although the changes in the tear film can be observed with a focal light source, ideally a blue light, the procedure is facilitated by slit-lamp biomicroscopy and a cobalt-blue filter. More readily available sources for a blue light include a Wood's lamp and the blue light on some models of direct ophthalmoscope.

Normal references ranges

Schirmer tear test (STT)

Dog   15–25 mm/min

Cat   3–32 mm/min. Low readings are expected in cats in the clinical setting; values should be
          interpreted with caution and in conjunction with clinical signs.

In both species a difference of >5 mm/min between the eyes is likely to be clinically relevant.

Intraocular pressure (IOP)

Dog   15–25 mmHg

Cat   15–25 mmHg

In both species a difference of >5 mmHg between the eyes is likely to be clinically relevant.

Tear film break-up time (TBUT)

Dog   approximately 20 s (range 15–25 s)

Cat   approximately 16 s (range 10–20 s)

Further Reading

Barnett, K.C., Sansom, J., Heinrich, C. (2002) *Canine Ophthalmology. An Atlas and Text*, W. B. Saunders, London, UK

Barnett, K.C., Crispin, S.M. (1998) *Feline Ophthalmology. An Atlas and Text*, W. B. Saunders, London, UK

de Lahunta, A. & Glass, E. (2009) *Veterinary Neuroanatomy and Clinical Neurology*, 3rd edn. Saunders Elsevier, St. Louis, Missouri, USA

Dubielzig, R.R., Ketring, K.L., McLellan, G.J., Daniel, A.M. (2010) *Veterinary Ocular Pathology: A Comparative Review*. Elsevier Health Sciences, USA

Forrester, J.V., Dick, A.D., McMenamin, P., Lee, R.L. (1996) *The Eye. Basic Sciences in Practice*, W. B. Saunders, London, UK

Gelatt, K.N. (2000) *Essentials of Veterinary Ophthalmology*, Lippincott Williams & Wilkins, Philadelphia, Pennsylvania, USA

Gelatt, K.N. (2007) *Veterinary Ophthalmology*, Blackwell Publishing, Iowa, USA

Gelatt, K.N., Gelatt, J.P. (2001) *Small Animal Ophthalmic Practical Techniques for the Veterinarian*, Butterworth-Heinemann, Oxford, UK

Grahn, B.H., Cullen, C.L., Peiffer, R.L. (2004) *Veterinary Ophthalmology Essentials*, Butterworth–Heinemann, Philadelphia, Pennsylvania, USA

Kaufman, P.A., Alm, A. (2002) *Adler's Physiology of the Eye*, 10th edn. Mosby Year Book, Inc., Missouri, USA

Maggs, D.J., Miller, P.E., Ofri, R. (2008) *Slatter's Fundamentals of Veterinary Ophthalmology*, 4th edn. Saunders Elsevier, Missouri, USA

Petersen-Jones, S.M., Crispin, S.M. (2002) *BSAVA Manual of Small Animal Ophthalmology*, 2nd edn. British Small Animal Veterinary Association, Gloucester, UK

Peiffer, R.L. Jr, Petersen Jones, S.M. (2001) *Small Animal Ophthalmology. A Problem-Orientated Approach*, 3rd edn. W.B. Saunders, London, UK

Penderis, J. (2004) Disorders of eyes and vision. In: *BSAVA Manual of Canine and Feline Neurology*, (eds S. Platt, N. Olby), 3rd edn. *British Small Animal Veterinary Association*, Gloucester, UK

Riis, R.C. (2002) *Small Animal Ophthalmology Secrets*, Hanley & Belfus, Inc., Philadelphia, Pennsylvania, USA

Glossary

This glossary provides the reader with definitions of ophthalmic terms used in the context of this book, and is not intended to be comprehensive.

Amaurosis (central blindness)	partial or total vision loss because of a lesion in the visual pathway excluding the eye
Anisocoria	unequal pupil size
Anterior chamber	region bounded anteriorly by the cornea and posteriorly by the plane of the iris and pupil
Anterior segment	all structures anterior to the face of the vitreous body
Aphakic crescent	crescent-shaped area between the equator of the lens and the margin of the pupil caused by a dislocated lens or by microphakia
Aqueous flare	scattering of light by protein and/or cells in the aqueous humour which occurs as a result of a breakdown of the blood-aqueous barrier; also known as Tyndall's phenomenon
Blepharospasm	spasm of the orbicularis oculi muscle resulting in involuntary closure of the eyelids
Blood-aqueous barrier	physical barrier at the level of the non-pigmented epithelium of the ciliary body and the endothelial cells of the iris vasculature
Bulbar conjunctiva	conjunctiva covering the globe
Buphthalmia/buphthalmos	enlargement of the globe (synonyms, hydrophthalmia, hydrophthalmos, megaloglobus)
Canaliculus	region of the nasolacrimal drainage system connecting the lacrimal punctum and the lacrimal sac
Canaliculops	cyst of the canaliculus
Canthus	anatomic region at the ends of the palpebral fissure where the upper and lower eyelids meet (medial canthus, lateral canthus)
Chemosis	conjunctival oedema
Ciliary flush	perilimbal redness caused by dilation of small blood vessels located at the limbus, e.g. in anterior uveitis (synonym, ciliary injection)

Small Animal Ophthalmology: What's Your Diagnosis? First Edition. Heidi Featherstone, Elaine Holt.
© 2011 by Heidi Featherstone and Elaine Holt. Published 2011 by Blackwell Publishing Ltd.

Cilium (pl. **cilia**)	eyelash
Coloboma	congenital absence of ocular tissue, e.g. eyelid coloboma
Conjunctivitis	inflammation of the conjunctiva
Consensual pupillary light reflex	see Appendix 1
Cycloplegia	paralysis of the ciliary body muscle resulting in loss of accommodation; usually accompanied by mydriasis
Cycloplegic	drug which induces cycloplegia, e.g. atropine
Dacryops	cyst within the lacrimal gland
Dazzle reflex	see Appendix 1
Desmarres chalazion clamp	surgical instrument consisting of a stainless-steel base plate and an opposing circular or oval ring; provides stabilization of the eyelid whilst allowing access
Direct pupillary light reflex	see Appendix 1
Distichium (pl. **distichia**)	extra eyelash that emerges from the meibomian gland orifice, posterior to the normal eyelashes; condition referred to as distichiasis
Dyscoria	irregular-shaped pupil
Ectopic cilium (pl. **cilia**)	extra eyelash which emerges through the palpebra conjunctiva from the region of the meibomian gland
Ectropion	outward turning of the eyelid and eyelid margin
Electroretinography	recording of retinal electrical potentials generated by light stimulation of the retina; includes the basic parameters, b-wave amplitude and latency. In the clinical setting it is most commonly employed to assess retinal function when the fundus is obscured by cataract, and in the differential diagnosis of blindness when the fundus appears normal.
Endophthalmitis	inflammation of the intraocular contents
Entropion	inward turning of the eyelid and eyelid margin towards the ocular surface
Enucleation	surgical removal of the globe and the eyelid margins, third eyelid and conjunctiva
Epiphora	overflow of tears
Episclera	superficial layer of the sclera
Episcleritis	inflammation of the episclera
Esotropia	convergent strabismus or medial deviation of the globe
Euryblepharon	abnormally large eyelid opening (synonym, macropalpebral fissure)

Exenteration	surgical removal of the entire contents of the orbit, including the eye
Exotropia	divergent strabismus or lateral deviation of the globe
Filtration angle	the angle created by the iris and the cornea (synonyms, anterior chamber angle, corneoiridociliary angle, iridocorneal angle)
Finnoff transilluminator	focal light source for examining the eye
Fundus	posterior portion of the eye as viewed through an ophthalmoscope; comprises retina, choroid, optic disc and sclera
Gland of Moll	modified apocrine sweat gland within the eyelid margin
Gland of Zeiss	sebaceous gland within the eyelid margin
Goniodysgenesis	the failure of rarefaction to form pectinate ligaments
Haab's striae	linear opacities in the cornea representative of breaks in Descemet's membrane, indicative of globe enlargement caused by glaucoma
Hemeralopia	day blindness
Heterochromia iridis	two or more colours in an iris or between two irides in one individual
High-frequency ultrasound biomicroscopy (HF-UBM)	ultrasound technique using frequencies between 50 and 100 MHz (higher than traditional B-mode ultrasound). Tissue resolution is increased approximately 10-fold compared with a 10 MHz probe.
Hotz-Celsus	surgical technique for correcting entropion
Hyaloid	pertaining to the vitreous
Hyphaema	haemorrhage in the anterior chamber
Hypotony	abnormally low intraocular pressure (usually <5 mmHg)
Indirect pupillary light reflex	see Appendix 1
Intracameral	within a chamber; used to describe an injection into the anterior chamber
Iridocorneal angle	the angle created by the iris and the cornea (synonyms, anterior chamber angle, filtration angle, corneoiridociliary angle)
Iridodonesis	tremulousness of the iris, usually associated with lens instability or lens removal
Iris collarette	junction between the central pupillary zone and the peripheral ciliary zone of the iris
Iris rest	dark brown/black focal deposit of uveal pigment on the anterior lens capsule; usually a sign of anterior uveitis
Keratectomy	excision of the cornea
Keratotomy	incision into the cornea

Keratic precipitates	aggregate of leucocytes adhering to the corneal endothelium
Keratitis	inflammation of the cornea
Keratoconjunctivitis sicca (KCS)	inflammation of the conjunctiva and cornea because of decreased aqueous tear production
Lacrimostimulant	drug that increases lacrimation
Lagophthalmos	inability to fully close the palpebral fissure
Leukocoria (leucokorea, leukocorea)	white pupil
Limbus	transitional zone between the cornea and the sclera
Macropalpebral fissure	abnormally large eyelid opening (synonym, euryblepharon)
Meibomian gland (tarsal gland)	sebaceous gland within the eyelid margin that produces meibum, the lipid component of the precorneal tear film
Microphakia	abnormally small lens
Mucinogenic	agent that stimulates the production of mucin (pertaining to the tear film)
Mucinometic	agent that simulates the presence of mucin in the tear film
Mydriasis	dilation of the pupil
Nuclear sclerosis	age-related hardening of the lens (synonym, lenticular sclerosis)
Nyctalopia	night blindness
Ophthalmoparesis	weakness of the ocular muscles
Ophthalmoplegia	paralysis of the ocular muscles
Optic disc	intraocular portion of the optic nerve in the eye (synonyms, optic papilla, optic nerve head)
Optic disc cupping	enlargement and deepening of the optic disc, most commonly following glaucoma ('glaucomatous cupping')
Palpebral conjunctiva	conjunctiva lining the eyelids and the third eyelid
Palpebral fissure	eyelid opening or aperture
Panophthalmitis	inflammation of all layers of the globe
Pectinate ligament dysplasia	term describing the gonioscopic view of the failure of rarefaction to form pectinate ligaments
Penetrating keratoplasty	full thickness corneal transplant
Peripapillary	surrounding the optic disc
Persistent pupillary membrane (PPM)	congenital remnant(s) of the prenatal pupillary vascular membrane; PPM remnants extend from the collarette of the iris to the cornea, lens, or other areas of the iris

Phacoclastic uveitis	severe proliferative inflammatory response as a result of rupture of the lens capsule
Phacodonesis	movement of the lens, usually secondary to partial breakdown of the lens zonules
Phacolytic uveitis	lymphocytic-plasmacytic inflammatory response secondary to the release of lens proteins through an intact lens capsule; commonly seen with developing cataracts and hypermature cataracts
Phthisis bulbi	atrophy of the globe with hypotony
Photopic	light or bright illumination conditions
Persistent hyperplastic primary vitreous (PHPV)	congenital anomaly in which the hyaloid vascular system persists in the adult eye
Pre-iridal fibrovascular membrane (PFIM)	fibrovascular membrane which forms on the anterior surface of the iris, most commonly seen on histopathology
Posterior capsular opacity	opacity of the posterior lens capsule and/or its remnant following surgical cataract extraction
Posterior chamber	space formed by the posterior surface of the iris and the anterior surface of the lens; contains aqueous humour
Posterior segment	portion of the eye comprising all the structures situated between the anterior face of the vitreous humour and the sclera
Posterior synechia (pl. synechiae)	adhesion between the pupil margin and the anterior lens capsule
Punctum	opening to the canaliculus of the nasolacrimal system
Purkinje image	see Appendix 1
Rose Bengal dye	topical ophthalmic stain used to assess the integrity of the tear film and to delineate corneal erosions
Rhytidectomy	excision of wrinkle
Rubeosis iridis	neovascularisation of the iris
Schirmer tear test (STT)	test used to assess aqueous tear production in mm/min; measures both basal and reflex tear production
Scleral venous plexus	network of veins in the sclera through which aqueous humour drains
Scotopic	dark or dim light conditions
Seidel test	assessment of corneal integrity by the observation of aqueous humour leakage following the application of fluorescein dye
Strabismus	deviation of the globe (synonym, heterotropia, squint)
Subalbinism	partial albinism, colour dilution, e.g. merle collie
Syneresis	liquefaction of the vitreous humour

Tapetal reflection (or reflex) see Appendix 1

Tarsorrhaphy surgical apposition of the eyelids

Tear film break-up time (TBUT) see Appendix 1

Tissue plasminogen activator (TPA) agent that causes the production of plasmin from plasminogen and in turn leads to the lysis of fibrin

Tropicamide parasympatholytic agent used as a short-acting mydriatic

Tunica vasculosa lentis network of blood vessels originating from the hyaloid artery and the iris which provide nutrition to the lens during development of the eye

Trichiasis hairs growing in a normal location, which contact the ocular surface

Index

Small Animal Ophthalmology: What's Your Diagnosis? First Edition. Heidi Featherstone, Elaine Holt.
© 2011 by Heidi Featherstone and Elaine Holt. Published 2011 by Blackwell Publishing Ltd.